Virtual Clinical Excursions—Pediatrics

for

James and Ashwill
Nursing Care of Children: Principles and Practice,
3rd Edition

Virtual Clinical Excursions—Pediatrics

for

James and Ashwill
Nursing Care of Children: Principles and Practice,
3rd Edition

prepared by

Betty W. Hamlisch, RN, MS Health Education
Professor of Nursing
Tompkins Cortland Community College
Dryden, New York

software developed by

Wolfsong Informatics, LLC
Tucson, Arizona

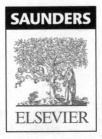

SAUNDERS

ELSEVIER

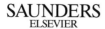

SAUNDERS
ELSEVIER

11830 Westline Industrial Dr.
St. Louis, Missouri 63146

VIRTUAL CLINICAL EXCURSIONS—PEDIATRICS FOR
JAMES AND ASHWILL
NURSING CARE OF CHILDREN: PRINCIPLES AND PRACTICE,
THIRD EDITION
Copyright © 2007 by Saunders, an imprint of Elsevier Inc.

ISBN-13: 978-1-4160-4458-1
ISBN-10: 1-4160-4458-2

All rights reserved. No part of this publication may be reproduced or transmitted in any form or by any means, electronic or mechanical, including photocopy, recording, or any information storage and retrieval system, without permission in writing from the publisher. Permissions may be sought directly from Elsevier's Rights Department in Philadelphia, PA, USA: phone: (+1) 215 239 3804, e-mail: healthpermissions@elsevier.com. You may also complete your request on-line via the Elsevier homepage (http://www.elsevier.com), by selecting "Customer Support" and then "Obtaining Permissions."

Although for mechanical reasons all pages of this publication are perforated, only those pages imprinted with a Elsevier Inc. copyright notice are intended for removal.

Notice

Knowledge and best practice in this field are constantly changing. As new research and experience broaden our knowledge, changes in practice, treatment and drug therapy may become necessary or appropriate. Readers are advised to check the most current information provided (i) on procedures featured or (ii) by the manufacturer of each product to be administered, to verify the recommended dose or formula, the method and duration of administration, and contraindications. It is the responsibility of the practitioner, relying on their own experience and knowledge of the patient, to make diagnoses, to determine dosages and the best treatment for each individual patient, and to take all appropriate safety precautions. To the fullest extent of the law, neither the Publisher nor the Authors assumes any liability for any injury and/or damage to persons or property arising out or related to any use of the material contained in this book.

ISBN-13: 978-1-4160-4458-1
ISBN-10: 1-4160-4458-2

Executive Editor: *Tom Wilhelm*
Managing Editor: *Jeff Downing*
Associate Developmental Editor: *Tiffany Trautwein*
Book Production Manager: *Gayle May*
Project Manager: *Tracey Schriefer*

Printed in the United States of America

Last digit is the print number: 9 8 7 6 5 4 3 2 1

Working together to grow
libraries in developing countries

www.elsevier.com | www.bookaid.org | www.sabre.org

ELSEVIER   BOOK AID International   Sabre Foundation

Workbook
prepared by

Betty W. Hamlisch, RN, MS Health Education
Professor of Nursing
Tompkins Cortland Community College
Dryden, New York

Textbook

Susan Rowen James, RN, PhD(c)
Associate Professor
Curry College Division of Nursing
Milton, Massachusetts

Jean Weiler Ashwill, MSN, RN
Director of Undergraduate Student Services
School of Nursing
University of Texas at Arlington
Arlington, Texas

Reviewer

Kelly Ann Crum, RN, MSN
Instructional Specialist
Lead Faculty
Curriculum Development/Maternal Child Nursing Specialty
Health Sciences and Nursing Department
University of Phoenix, Online
Phoenix, Arizona

Contents

Getting Started

Getting Set Up 1

A Quick Tour 9

A Detailed Tour 24

Reducing Medication Errors 37

Unit 1—Carrie Richards

Lesson 1   The Hospitalized Infant (Chapters 4, 5, and 11) 43

Lesson 2   Caring for an Infant with Bronchiolitis (Chapters 5, 13, and 21) 51

Lesson 3   Nursing Care Issues Associated with Bronchiolitis (Chapters 14, 18, and 21) 63

Lesson 4   Caring for an Infant Who Is Failing to Thrive (Chapters 4, 5, and 29) 77

Unit 2—Stephanie Brown

Lesson 5   The Young Child in the Hospital (Chapters 4, 6, and 11) 87

Lesson 6   Caring for a Young Child with Meningitis (Chapters 13 and 28) 97

Lesson 7   Caring for a Young Child with Cerebral Palsy (Chapters 4 and 28) 109

Unit 3—George Gonzalez

Lesson 8   The Hospitalized School-Age Child (Chapters 4, 7, and 11) 119

Lesson 9   Caring for a School-Age Child with Diabetes Mellitus (Chapter 27) 127

Lesson 10   Teaching Self-Care to a Child with Diabetes and His Family (Chapter 27) ... 141

Unit 4—Tiffany Sheldon

Lesson 11   The Hospitalized Adolescent (Chapters 8 and 11) 151

Lesson 12   Caring for a Teen with an Eating Disorder: Part 1 (Chapter 29) 159

Lesson 13   Caring for a Teen with an Eating Disorder: Part 2 (Chapter 29) 167

Unit 5—Tommy Douglas

Lesson 14   Caring for a Child and Family in the Emergency Department
(Chapters 10 and 28) 177

Lesson 15   Emergency Care for a Child with a Head Injury (Chapter 28) 185

Lesson 16   Providing Support for Families Experiencing the Loss of a Child
(Chapters 1 and 12) 193

Unit 6—Nursing Care of Infants and Children

Lesson 17   Safety for Infants and Young Children (Chapters 4, 5, 6, 7, and 8) 201

Lesson 18   Medication Administration in Children (Chapter 14) 213

Lesson 19   Pediatric Nursing Care Management: Part 1
(Chapters 11, 12, 21, 27, 28, and 29) 223

Lesson 20   Pediatric Nursing Care Management: Part 2
(Chapters 11, 12, 21, 27, 28, 29, and 30) 233

Table of Contents
James and Ashwill
Nursing Care of Children: Principles and Practice, 3rd Edition

Unit I Introduction to Child Health Nursing

1 Foundations of Child Health Nursing (Lesson 16)

Unit II Growth and Development: The Child and the Family

2 Family-Centered Nursing Care
3 Communicating with Children and Families
4 Health Promotion for the Developing Child (Lessons 1, 4, 5, 7, 8, and 17)
5 Health Promotion for the Infant (Lessons 1, 2, 4, and 17)
6 Health Promotion During Early Childhood (Lessons 5 and 17)
7 Health Promotion for the School-Age Child (Lessons 8 and 17)
8 Health Promotion for the Adolescent (Lessons 11 and 17)

Unit III Special Considerations in Caring for Children

9 Physical Assessment of Children
10 Emergency Care of the Child (Lesson 14)
11 The Ill Child in the Hospital and Other Care Settings (Lessons 1, 5, 8, 11, 19, and 20)
12 The Child with a Chronic Condition or Terminal Illness (Lessons 16, 19, and 20)
13 Principles and Procedures for Nursing Care of Children (Lessons 2 and 6)
14 Medicating Infants and Children (Lessons 3 and 18)
15 Pain Management for Children

Unit IV Caring for Children with Health Problems

16 The Child with an Infectious Disease
17 The Child with an Immunologic Alteration
18 The Child with a Fluid and Electrolyte Alteration (Lesson 3)
19 The Child with a Gastrointestinal Alteration
20 The Child with a Genitourinary Alteration
21 The Child with a Respiratory Alteration (Lessons 2, 3, 19, and 20)
22 The Child with a Cardiovascular Alteration
23 The Child with a Hematologic Alteration
24 The Child with Cancer
25 The Child with an Integumentary Alteration
26 The Child with a Musculoskeletal Alteration
27 The Child with an Endocrine or Metabolic Alteration (Lessons 9, 10, 19, and 20)
28 The Child with a Neurologic Alteration (Lessons 6, 7, 14, 15, 19, and 20)
29 The Child with a Psychosocial Disorder (Lessons 4, 12, 13, 19, and 20)
30 The Child with a Cognitive Impairment (Lesson 20)
31 The Child with a Sensory Alteration

Appendixes

A Recommendations for Preventive Pediatric Health Care
B Growth Charts
C Normal Blood Pressure Readings for Children

Getting Started

GETTING SET UP

■ MINIMUM SYSTEM REQUIREMENTS

WINDOWS™

Windows XP, 2000, 98, ME, NT 4.0 (Recommend Windows XP/2000)
Pentium® III processor (or equivalent) @ 600 MHz (Recommend 800 MHz or better)
128 MB of RAM (Recommend 256 MB or more)
800 x 600 screen size (Recommend 1024 x 768)
Thousands of colors
12x CD-ROM drive
Soundblaster 16 soundcard compatibility
Stereo speakers or headphones

Note: Virtual Clinical Excursions—Pediatrics for Windows will require a minimal amount of disk space to install icons and required dll files for Windows 98/ME.

MACINTOSH®

MAC OS X (10.2 or higher)
Apple Power PC G3 @ 500 MHz or better
128 MB of RAM (Recommend 256 MB or more)
800 x 600 screen size (Recommend 1024 x 768)
Thousands of colors
12x CD-ROM drive
Stereo speakers or headphones

1

Copyright © 2007 by Saunders, an imprint of Elsevier Inc. All rights reserved.

■ INSTALLATION INSTRUCTIONS

WINDOWS

1. Insert the *Virtual Clinical Excursions—Pediatrics* CD-ROM.
2. Inserting the CD should automatically bring up the setup screen if the current product is not already installed.
    a. If the setup screen does not appear automatically (and *Virtual Clinical Excursions—Pediatrics* has not been installed already), navigate to the "My Computer" icon on your desktop or in your Start menu.
    b. Double-click on your CD-ROM drive.
    c. If installation does not start at this point:
        (1) Click the **Start** icon on the task bar and select the **Run** option.
        (2) Type d:\setup.exe (where "d:\" is your CD-ROM drive) and press **OK**.
        (3) Follow the onscreen instructions for installation.
3. Follow the onscreen instructions during the setup process.

MACINTOSH

1. Insert the *Virtual Clinical Excursions—Pediatrics* CD in the CD-ROM drive. The disk icon will appear on your desktop.

2. Double-click on the disk icon.

3. Double-click on the PEDIATRICS_MAC run file.

Note: Virtual Clinical Excursions—Pediatrics for Macintosh does not have an installation setup and can only be run directly from the CD.

■ HOW TO USE VIRTUAL CLINICAL EXCURSIONS—PEDIATRICS

WINDOWS

1. Double-click on the *Virtual Clinical Excursions—Pediatrics* icon located on your desktop.
2. Or navigate to the program via the Windows Start menu.

Note: Windows 98/ME will require you to restart your computer before running the *Virtual Clinical Excursions—Pediatrics* program.

MACINTOSH

1. Insert the *Virtual Clinical Excursions—Pediatrics* CD in the CD-ROM drive. The disk icon will appear on your desktop.

2. Double-click on the disk icon.

3. Double-click on the PEDIATRICS_MAC run file.

Copyright © 2007 by Saunders, an imprint of Elsevier Inc. All rights reserved.

■ SCREEN SETTINGS

For best results, your computer monitor resolution should be set at a minimum of 800 x 600. The number of colors displayed should be set to "thousands or higher" (High Color or 16 bit) or "millions of colors" (True Color or 24 bit).

Windows™

1. From the **Start** menu, select **Control Panel** (on some systems, you will first go to **Settings**, then to **Control Panel**).
2. Double-click on the **Display** icon.
3. Click on the **Settings** tab.
4. Under **Screen resolution** use the slider bar to select **800 by 600 pixels**.
5. Access the **Colors** drop-down menu by clicking on the down arrow.
6. Select **High Color (16 bit)** or **True Color (24 bit)**.
7. Click on **OK**.
8. You may be asked to verify the setting changes. Click **Yes**.
9. You may be asked to restart your computer to accept the changes. Click **Yes**.

Macintosh®

1. Select the **Monitors** control panel.
2. Select **800 x 600** (or similar) from the **Resolution** area.
3. Select **Thousands** or **Millions** from the **Color Depth** area.

■ WEB BROWSERS

Supported web browsers include Microsoft Internet Explorer (IE) version 6.0 or higher, Netscape version 7.1 or higher, and Mozilla Firefox 1.4 or higher.

If you use America Online (AOL) for web access, you will need AOL version 4.0 or higher. Do not use earlier versions of AOL with earlier versions of IE, because you will have difficulty accessing many features.

For best results with AOL:
- Connect to the Internet using AOL version 4.0 or higher.
- Open a private chat within AOL (this allows the AOL client to remain open, without asking whether you wish to disconnect while minimized).
- Minimize AOL.
- Launch a recommended browser.

■ TECHNICAL SUPPORT

Technical support for this product is available between 7:30 a.m. and 7 p.m. (CST), Monday through Friday. Before calling, be sure that your computer meets the minimum system requirements to run this software. Inside the United States and Canada, call 1-800-692-9010. Outside North America, call 314-872-8370. You may also fax your questions to 314-523-4932 or contact Technical Support through e-mail: technical.support@elsevier.com.

Trademarks: Windows, Macintosh, Pentium, and America Online are registered trademarks.

Copyright © 2007 by Mosby, Inc., an affiliate of Elsevier Inc.

All rights reserved. No part of this product may be reproduced or transmitted in any form or by any means, electronic or mechanical, including input or storage in any information system, without written permission from the publisher.

Copyright © 2007 by Saunders, an imprint of Elsevier Inc. All rights reserved.

ACCESSING *Virtual Clinical Excursions—Pediatrics* FROM EVOLVE

The product you have purchased is part of the Evolve family of online courses and learning resources. Please read the following information thoroughly to get started.

To access your instructor's course on Evolve:

Your instructor will provide you with the username and password needed to access this specific course on the Evolve Learning System. Once you have received this information, please follow these instructions:

1. Go to the Evolve student page (http://evolve.elsevier.com/student)

2. Enter your username and password in the **Login to My Evolve** area and click the **Login** button.

3. You will be taken to your personalized **My Evolve** page, where the course will be listed in the **My Courses** module.

TECHNICAL REQUIREMENTS

To use an Evolve course, you will need access to a computer that is connected to the Internet and equipped with web browser software that supports frames. For optimal performance, it is recommended that you have speakers and use a high-speed Internet connection. However, slower dial-up modems (56 K minimum) are acceptable.

Copyright © 2007 by Saunders, an imprint of Elsevier Inc. All rights reserved.

Whichever browser you use, the browser preferences must be set to enable cookies and JavaScript and the cache must be set to reload every time.

Enable Cookies

Browser	Steps
Internet Explorer (IE) 6.0 or higher	1. Select **Tools → Internet Options**. 2. Select **Privacy** tab. 3. Use the slider (slide down) to **Accept All Cookies**. 4. Click **OK**. -OR- 3. Click the **Advanced** button. 4. Click the check box next to **Override Automatic Cookie Handling**. 5. Click the **Accept** buttons under **First-party Cookies** and **Third-party Cookies**. 6. Click **OK**.
Netscape 7.1 or higher	1. Select **Edit → Preferences**. 2. Select **Privacy & Security**. 3. Select **Cookies**. 4. Select **Enable All Cookies**.
Mozilla Firefox 1.4 or higher	1. Select **Tools → Options**. 2. Select **Privacy** icon. 3. Click to expand Cookies. 4. Select **Allow sites to set cookies**. 5. Click **OK**.

Copyright © 2007 by Saunders, an imprint of Elsevier Inc. All rights reserved.

Enable JavaScript

Browser	Steps
Internet Explorer (IE) 6.0 or higher	1. Select **Tools → Internet Options**. 2. Select **Security** tab. 3. Under **Security level for this zone** set to **Medium** or lower.
Netscape 7.1 or higher	1. Select **Edit → Preferences**. 2. Select **Advanced**. 3. Select **Scripts & Plugins**. 4. Make sure the **Navigator** box is checked to **Enable JavaScript**. 5. Click **OK**.
Mozilla Firefox 1.4 or higher	1. Select **Tools → Options**. 2. Select the **Content** icon. 3. Select **Enable JavaScript**. 4. Click **OK**.

Set Cache to Always Reload a Page

Browser	Steps
Internet Explorer (IE) 6.0 or higher	1. Select **Tools → Internet Options**. 2. Select **General** tab. 3. Go to the **Temporary Internet Files** and click the **Settings** button. 4. Select the radio button for **Every visit to the page** and click **OK** when complete.
Netscape 7.1 or higher	1. Select **Edit → Preferences**. 2. Select **Advanced**. 3. Select **Cache**. 4. Select the **Every time I view the page** radio button. 5. Click **OK**.
Mozilla Firefox 1.4 or higher	1. Select **Tools → Options**. 2. Select the **Privacy** icon. 3. Click to expand Cache. 4. Set the value to "**0**" in the **Use up to: ___ MB of disk space for the cache** field. 5. Click **OK**.

Copyright © 2007 by Saunders, an imprint of Elsevier Inc. All rights reserved.

Plug-Ins

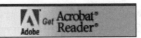
Adobe Acrobat Reader—With the free Acrobat Reader software, you can view and print Adobe PDF files. Many Evolve products offer student and instructor manuals, checklists, and more in this format!

Download at: http://www.adobe.com

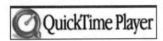
Apple QuickTime—Install this to hear word pronunciations, heart and lung sounds, and many other helpful audio clips within Evolve Online Courses!

Download at: http://www.apple.com

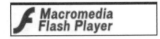
Macromedia Flash Player—This player will enhance your viewing of many Evolve web pages, as well as educational short-form to long-form animation within the Evolve Learning System!

Download at: http://www.macromedia.com

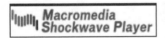
Macromedia Shockwave Player—Shockwave is best for viewing the many interactive learning activities within Evolve Online Courses!

Download at: http://www.macromedia.com

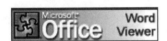
Microsoft Word Viewer—With this viewer Microsoft Word users can share documents with those who don't have Word, and users without Word can open and view Word documents. Many Evolve products have testbank, student and instructor manuals, and other documents available for downloading and viewing on your own computer!

Download at: http://www.microsoft.com

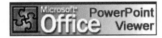
Microsoft PowerPoint Viewer—View PowerPoint 97, 2000, and 2002 presentations even if you don't have PowerPoint with this viewer. Many Evolve products have slides available for downloading and viewing on your own computer!

Download at: http://www.microsoft.com

Copyright © 2007 by Saunders, an imprint of Elsevier Inc. All rights reserved.

SUPPORT INFORMATION

Live support is available to customers in the United States and Canada from 7:30 a.m. to 7 p.m. (CST), Monday through Friday by calling **1-800-401-9962**. You can also send an email to evolve-support@elsevier.com.

There is also **24/7 support information** available on the Evolve website (http://evolve.elsevier.com), including:

- Guided Tours
- Tutorials
- Frequently Asked Questions (FAQs)
- Online Copies of Course User Guides
- And much more!

Copyright © 2007 by Saunders, an imprint of Elsevier Inc. All rights reserved.

A QUICK TOUR

Welcome to *Virtual Clinical Excursions—Pediatrics*, a virtual hospital setting in which you can work with multiple complex patient simulations and also learn to access and evaluate the information resources that are essential for high-quality patient care.

The virtual hospital, Pacific View Regional Hospital, has realistic architecture and access to patient rooms, a Nurses' Station, and a Medication Room.

■ BEFORE YOU START

Make sure you have your textbook nearby when you use the *Virtual Clinical Excursions—Pediatrics* CD. You will want to consult topic areas in your textbook frequently while working with the CD and using this workbook.

■ HOW TO SIGN IN

- Enter your name on the Student Nurse identification badge.
- Now choose one of the four periods of care in which to work. In Periods of Care 1 through 3, you can actively engage in patient assessment, entry of data in the electronic patient record (EPR), and medication administration. Period of Care 4 presents the day in review. Highlight and click the appropriate period of care. (For this quick tour, choose **Period of Care 1: 0730-0815**.)
- This takes you to the Patient List screen (see example on page 11). Only the patients on the Pediatrics Floor are available. Note that the virtual time is provided in the box at the lower left corner of the screen (0731, since we chose Period of Care 1).

Note: If you choose to work during Period of Care 4: 1900-2000, the Patient List screen is skipped since you are not able to visit patients or administer medications during the shift. Instead, you are taken directly to the Nurses' Station, where the records of all the patients on the floor are available for your review.

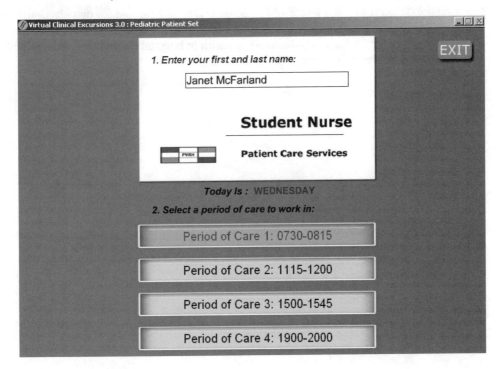

Copyright © 2007 by Saunders, an imprint of Elsevier Inc. All rights reserved.

■ **PATIENT LIST**

PEDIATRICS UNIT

George Gonzalez (Room 301)
Diabetic ketoacidosis—An 11-year-old Hispanic male admitted for stabilization of blood glucose level and diabetic re-education associated with his diagnosis of type 1 diabetes mellitus. This patient's poor compliance with insulin therapy and dietary regime have resulted in frequent and repeated hospital admissions for DKA.

Tommy Douglas (Room 302)
Traumatic brain injury—A 6-year-old Caucasian male transferred from the Pediatric Intensive Care Unit in preparation for organ donation. This patient is status post ventriculostomy with negative intracerebral blood flow and requires extensive hemodynamic monitoring and support, along with compassionate family care.

Carrie Richards (Room 303)
Bronchiolitis—A 3½-month-old African-American female admitted with respiratory distress due to respiratory syncytial virus, along with dehydration and a poor nutritional status. Parent education and support are among her primary needs.

Stephanie Brown (Room 304)
Meningitis—A 3-year-old African-American female with a history of spastic cerebral palsy admitted for intravenous antibiotic therapy, neurologic monitoring, and support for a diagnosis of acute meningitis. Maintenance of physical and occupational programs addressing her mobility limitations complicate her acute care stay.

Tiffany Sheldon (Room 305)
Anorexia nervosa—A 14-year-old Caucasian female admitted for dehydration, electrolyte imbalance, and malnutrition following a syncope episode at home. This patient has a history of eating disorders, which have resulted in multiple hospital admissions and strained family dynamics between mother and daughter.

Copyright © 2007 by Saunders, an imprint of Elsevier Inc. All rights reserved.

■ HOW TO SELECT A PATIENT

- You can choose one or more patients to work with from the Patient List by checking the box to the left of the patient name(s). For this quick tour, select Stephanie Brown. (In order to receive a scorecard for a patient, the patient must be selected before proceeding to the Nurses' Station.)
- Click on **Get Report** to the right of the medical records number (MRN) to view a summary of the patient's care during the 12-hour period before your arrival on the unit.
- After reviewing the report, click on **Go to Nurses' Station** in the right lower corner to begin your care. (*Note:* If you have been assigned to care for multiple patients, you can click on **Return to Patient List** to select and review the report for each additional patient before going to the Nurses' Station.)

Note: Even though the Patient List is initially skipped when you sign in to work for Period of Care 4, you can still access this screen if you wish to review the shift-change report for any of the patients. To do so, simply click on **Patient List** near the top left corner of the Nurses' Station (or click on the clipboard to the left of the Kardex). Then click on **Get Report** for the patient(s) whose care you are reviewing. This may be done during any period of care.

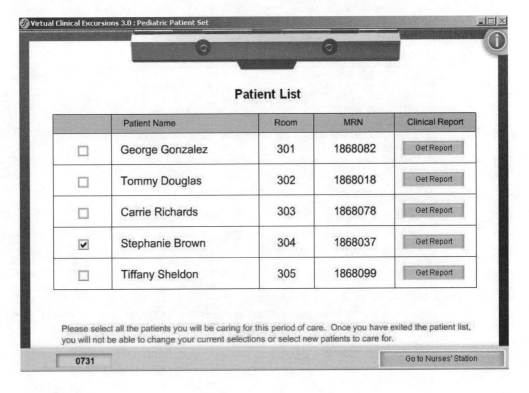

Copyright © 2007 by Saunders, an imprint of Elsevier Inc. All rights reserved.

■ HOW TO FIND A PATIENT'S RECORDS

NURSES' STATION

Within the Nurses' Station, you will see:

1. A clipboard that contains the patient list for that floor.
2. A chart rack with patient charts labeled by room number, a notebook labeled Kardex, and a notebook labeled MAR (Medication Administration Record).
3. A desktop computer with access to the Electronic Patient Record (EPR).
4. A tool bar across the top of the screen that can also be used to access the Patient List, EPR, Chart, MAR, and Kardex. This tool bar is also accessible from each patient's room.
5. A Drug Guide containing information about the medications you are able to administer to your patients.
6. A tool bar across the bottom of the screen that you can use to access patient rooms, the Medication Room, the Floor Map, or the Drug Guide.

As you run your cursor over an item, it will be highlighted. To select, simply double-click on the item. As you use these resources, you will always be able to return to the Nurses' Station by clicking on the **Return to Nurses' Station** bar located in the right lower corner of your screen.

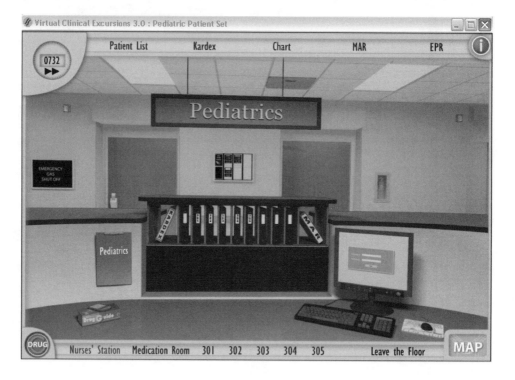

Copyright © 2007 by Saunders, an imprint of Elsevier Inc. All rights reserved.

MEDICATION ADMINISTRATION RECORD (MAR)

The MAR icon located in the tool bar at the top of your screen accesses current 24-hour medications for each patient. Click on the icon and the MAR will open. (*Note:* You can also access the MAR by clicking on the MAR notebook on the far right side of the book rack in the center of the screen.) Within the MAR, tabs on the right side of the screen allow you to select patients by room number. Be careful to make sure you select the correct tab number for *your* patient rather than simply reading the first record that appears after the MAR opens. Each MAR sheet lists the following:

- Medications
- Route and dosage of each medication
- Times of administration of each medication

Note: The MAR changes each day. Expired MARs are stored in the patients' charts.

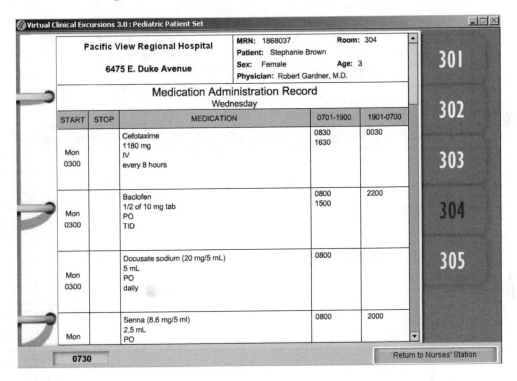

Copyright © 2007 by Saunders, an imprint of Elsevier Inc. All rights reserved.

CHARTS

To access patient charts, either click on the **Chart** icon at the top of your screen or anywhere within the chart rack in the center of the Nurses' Station screen. When the close-up view appears, the individual charts are labeled by room number. To open a chart, click on the room number of the patient whose chart you wish to review. The patient's name and allergies will appear on the left side of the screen, along with a list of tabs on the right side of the screen, allowing you to view the following data:

- Allergies
- Physician's Orders
- Physician's Notes
- Nurse's Notes
- Laboratory Reports
- Diagnostic Reports
- Surgical Reports
- Consultations

- Patient Education
- History and Physical
- Nursing Admission
- Expired MARs
- Consents
- Mental Health
- Admissions
- Emergency Department

Information appears in real time. The entries are in reverse chronologic order, so use the down arrow at the right side of each chart page to scroll down to view previous entries. Flip from tab to tab to view multiple data fields or click on the **Return to Nurses' Station** bar in the lower right corner of the screen to exit the chart.

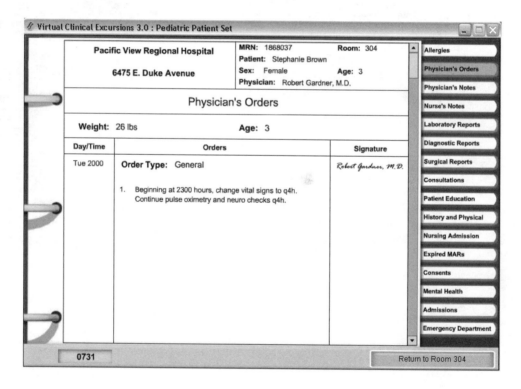

Copyright © 2007 by Saunders, an imprint of Elsevier Inc. All rights reserved.

ELECTRONIC PATIENT RECORD (EPR)

The EPR can be accessed from the computer in the Nurses' Station or from the EPR icon located in the tool bar at the top of your screen. To access a patient's EPR:

- Click on either the computer screen or the **EPR** icon.
- Your username and password are automatically filled in.
- Click on **Login** to enter the EPR.
- *Note:* Like the MAR, the EPR is arranged numerically. Thus when you enter, you are initially shown the records of the patient in the lowest room number on the floor. To view the correct data for *your* patient, remember to select the correct room number, using the drop-down menu for the Patient field at the top left corner of the screen.

The EPR used in Pacific View Regional Hospital represents a composite of commercial versions being used in hospitals. You can access the EPR:

- to review existing data for a patient (by room number).
- to enter data you collect while working with a patient.

The EPR is updated daily, so no matter what day or part of a shift you are working, there will be a current EPR with the patient's data from the past days of the current hospital stay. This type of simulated EPR allows you to examine how data for different attributes have changed over time, as well as to examine data for all of a patient's attributes at a particular time. The EPR is fully functional (as it is in a real-life hospital). You can enter such data as blood pressure, breath sounds, and certain treatments. The EPR will not, however, allow you to enter data for a previous time period. Use the arrows at the bottom of the screen to move forward and backward in time.

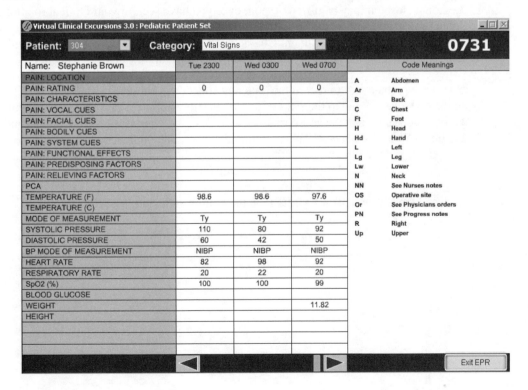

Name: Stephanie Brown	Tue 2300	Wed 0300	Wed 0700	Code Meanings	
PAIN: LOCATION				A	Abdomen
PAIN: RATING	0	0	0	Ar	Arm
PAIN: CHARACTERISTICS				B	Back
PAIN: VOCAL CUES				C	Chest
PAIN: FACIAL CUES				Ft	Foot
PAIN: BODILY CUES				H	Head
PAIN: SYSTEM CUES				Hd	Hand
PAIN: FUNCTIONAL EFFECTS				L	Left
PAIN: PREDISPOSING FACTORS				Lg	Leg
PAIN: RELIEVING FACTORS				Lw	Lower
PCA				N	Neck
TEMPERATURE (F)	98.6	98.6	97.6	NN	See Nurses notes
TEMPERATURE (C)				OS	Operative site
MODE OF MEASUREMENT	Ty	Ty	Ty	Or	See Physicians orders
SYSTOLIC PRESSURE	110	80	92	PN	See Progress notes
DIASTOLIC PRESSURE	60	42	50	R	Right
BP MODE OF MEASUREMENT	NIBP	NIBP	NIBP	Up	Upper
HEART RATE	82	98	92		
RESPIRATORY RATE	20	22	20		
SpO2 (%)	100	100	99		
BLOOD GLUCOSE					
WEIGHT			11.82		
HEIGHT					

Patient: 304   Category: Vital Signs   0731

Exit EPR

Copyright © 2007 by Saunders, an imprint of Elsevier Inc. All rights reserved.

At the top of the EPR screen, you can choose patients by their room numbers. In addition, you have access to 17 different categories of patient data. To change patients or data categories, click the down arrow to the right of the room number or category.

The categories of patient data in the EPR as as follows:

- Vital Signs
- Respiratory
- Cardiovascular
- Neurologic
- Gastrointestinal
- Excretory
- Musculoskeletal
- Integumentary
- Reproductive
- Psychosocial
- Wounds and Drains
- Activity
- Hygiene and Comfort
- Safety
- Nutrition
- IV
- Intake and Output

Remember, each hospital selects its own codes. The codes used in the EPR at Pacific View Regional Hospital may be different from ones you have seen in your clinical rotations. Take some time to acquaint yourself with the codes. Within the Vital Signs category, click on any item in the left column (e.g., Pain: Characteristics). In the far-right column, you will see a list of code meanings for the possible findings and/or descriptors for that assessment area.

You will use the codes to record the data you collect as you work with patients. Click on the box in the last time column to the right of any item and wait for the code meanings applicable to that entry to appear. Select the appropriate code to describe your assessment findings and type it in the box. (*Note:* If no cursor appears within the box, click on the box again until the blue shading disappears and the blinking cursor appears.) Once the data are typed in this box, they are entered into the patient's record for this period of care only.

To leave the EPR, click on **Exit EPR** in the bottom right corner of the screen.

Copyright © 2007 by Saunders, an imprint of Elsevier Inc. All rights reserved.

■ **VISITING A PATIENT**

From the Nurses' Station, click on the room number of the patient you wish to visit in the tool bar at the bottom of your screen. Once you are inside the room, you will see a still photo of your patient in the top left corner. To verify that this is the patient you have chosen, click on the **Check Armband** icon to the right of the photo. The patient's identification data will appear. If you click on **Check Allergies** (the next icon to the right), a list of the patient's allergies (if any) will replace the photo.

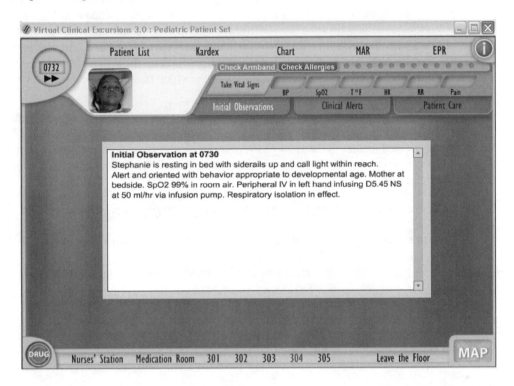

Also located in the patient's room are multiple icons you can use to assess the patient or the patient's medications. A virtual clock is provided in the upper left corner of the room to monitor your progress in real time. (*Note:* The fast-forward icon within the virtual clock will advance the time by 2-minute intervals when clicked.)

- The tool bar across the top of the screen allows you to check the **Patient List**, access the **EPR** to check or enter data, and view the patient's **Chart**, **MAR**, or **Kardex**.

- The **Take Vital Signs** icon allows you to measure the patient's up-to-the-minute blood pressure, oxygen saturation, temperature, heart rate, respiratory rate, and pain level.

- Each time you enter a patient's room, you are given an Initial Observation report to review (in the text box under the patient's photo). These notes are provided to give you a "look" at the patient as if you had just stepped into the room. You can also click on the **Initial Observations** icon to return to this box from other views within the patient's room. To the right of this icon is **Clinical Alerts**, a resource that allows you to make decisions about priority medication interventions based on emerging data collected in real time. Check this screen throughout your period of care to avoid missing critical information related to recently ordered or STAT medications.

- Clicking on the **Patient Care** icon opens up three specific learning environments within the patient room: **Physical Assessment**, **Nurse-Client Interactions**, and **Medication Administration**.

- To perform a **Physical Assessment**, choose a body area (such as **Head & Neck**) by clicking on the appropriate icon in the column of yellow buttons. This activates a list of system subcategories for that body area (e.g., see **Sensory**, **Neurologic**, etc. in the green boxes). After

Copyright © 2007 by Saunders, an imprint of Elsevier Inc. All rights reserved.

you click on the system that you wish to evaluate, a still photo and text box appear, describing the assessment findings. The still photo is a "snapshot" of how an assessment of this area might be done or what the finding might look like. For every body area, there is also an **Equipment** button located on the far right of the screen.

- To the right of the Physical Assessment icon is **Nurse-Client Interactions**. Clicking on this icon will reveal the times and titles of any videos available for viewing. (*Note:* If the video you wish to see is not listed, this means you have not yet reached the correct virtual time to view that video. Check the virtual clock; you may return to access the video once its designated time has occurred—as long as you do so within the same period of care. Or you can click on the fast-forward icon within the virtual clock to advance the time by 2-minute intervals. You will then need to click again on **Patient Care** and **Nurse-Client Interactions** to refresh the screen.) To view a listed video, click on the white arrow to the right of the video title. Use the control buttons below the video to start, stop, pause, rewind, or fast-forward the action or to mute the sound.

- **Medication Administration** is the pathway that allows you to review and administer medications to a patient after you have prepared them in the Medication Room. This process is addressed further in the *How to Prepare Medications* section (pages 19-20) and in *Medications* (pages 26-30). For additional hands-on practice, see *Reducing Medication Errors* (pages 37-41).

■ **HOW TO QUIT, CHANGE PATIENTS, OR CHANGE PERIOD OF CARE**

How to Quit: From most screens, you may click the **Leave the Floor** icon on the bottom tool bar to the right of the patient room numbers. (*Note:* From some screens, you will first need to click an **Exit** button or **Return to Nurses' Station** before clicking **Leave the Floor**.) When the Floor Menu appears, click **Exit** to leave the program.

How to Change Patients or Period of Care: To change patients, simply click on the new patient's room number. (You cannot receive a scorecard for a new patient, however, unless you have already selected that patient on the Patient List screen.) To change to a new period of care or to restart the virtual clock, click on **Leave the Floor** and then on **Restart the Program**.

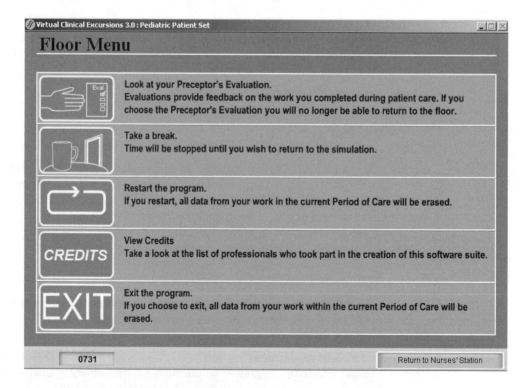

Copyright © 2007 by Saunders, an imprint of Elsevier Inc. All rights reserved.

■ HOW TO PREPARE MEDICATIONS

From the Nurses' Station or the patient's room, you can access the Medication Room by clicking on the icon in the tool bar at the bottom of your screen to the left of the patient room numbers.

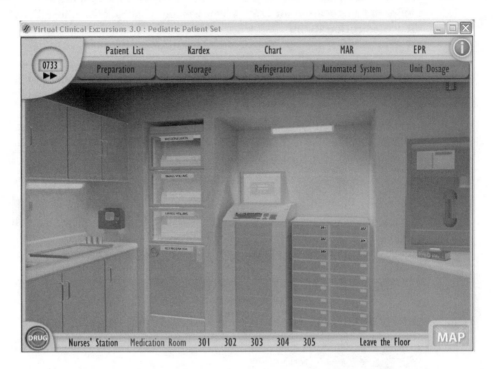

In the Medication Room you have access to the following (from left to right):

- A preparation area is located on the counter under the cabinets. To begin the medication preparation process, click on the tray on the counter or click on the **Preparation** icon at the top of the screen. The next screen leads you through a specific sequence (called the Preparation Wizard) to prepare medications one at a time for administration to a patient. However, no medication has been selected at this time. We will do this while working with a patient in *A Detailed Tour*. To exit this screen, click on **View Medication Room**.

- To the right of the cabinets (and above the refrigerator), IV storage bins are provided. Click on the bins themselves or on the **IV Storage** icon at the top of the screen. The bins are labeled **Microinfusion**, **Small Volume**, and **Large Volume**. Click on an individual bin to see a list of its contents. If you needed to prepare an IV medication at this time, you could click on the medication and its label would appear to the right under the patient's name. Next, you would click **Put Medication on Tray**. If you ever change your mind or choose the incorrect medication, you can reverse your actions by clicking on **Put Medication in Bin**. Click **Close Bin** in the right bottom corner to exit. **View Medication Room** brings you back to a full view of the entire room.

- A refrigerator is located under the IV storage bins to hold any medications that must be stored below room temperature. Click on the refrigerator door or on the **Refrigerator** icon at the top of the screen. Then click on the close-up view of the door to access the medications. When you are finished, click **Close Door** and then **View Medication Room**.

Copyright © 2007 by Saunders, an imprint of Elsevier Inc. All rights reserved.

- To prepare controlled substances, click the **Automated System** icon at the top of the screen or click the computer monitor located to the right of the IV storage bins. A login screen will appear; your name and password are automatically filled in. Click **Login**. Select the patient for whom you wish to access medications; then select the correct medication drawer to open (they are stored alphabetically). Click **Open Drawer**, highlight the proper medication, and choose **Put Medication on Tray**. When you are finished, click **Close Drawer** and then **View Medication Room**.

- Next to the Automated System is a set of drawers identified by patient room number. To access these, click on the drawers themselves or on the **Unit Dosage** icon at the top of the screen. This provides a close-up view of the drawers. To open a drawer, click on the room number of the patient you are working with. Next, click on the medication you would like to prepare for the patient, and a label will appear to the right, listing the medication strength, units, and dosage per unit. You can **Open** and **Close** this medication label by clicking the appropriate icon. To exit, click **Close Drawer**; then click **View Medication Room**.

At any time, you can learn about a medication you wish to prepare for a patient by clicking on the **Drug** icon in the bottom left corner of the medication room screen or by clicking the **Drug Guide** book on the counter to the right of the unit dosage drawers. The **Drug Guide** provides information about the medications commonly included in nursing drug handbooks. Nutritional supplements and maintenance intravenous fluid preparations are not included.

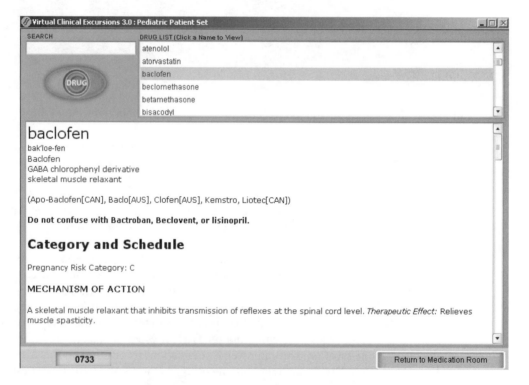

To access the MAR to review the medications ordered for a patient, click on the **MAR** icon located in the tool bar at the top of your screen and then click on the correct tab for your patient's room number. You may also click the **Review MAR** icon in the tool bar at the bottom of your screen from inside each medication storage area.

After you have chosen and prepared your medications, return to the patient's room to administer them by clicking on the room number in the bottom tool bar. Once inside the patient's room, click on **Patient Care** and then on **Medication Administration** and follow the proper administration sequence.

Copyright © 2007 by Saunders, an imprint of Elsevier Inc. All rights reserved.

■ **PRECEPTOR'S EVALUATIONS**

When you have finished a session, click on **Leave the Floor** to go to the Floor Menu. At this point, you can click on the top icon (**Look at Your Preceptor's Evaluation**) to receive a score-card that provides feedback on the work you completed during patient care.

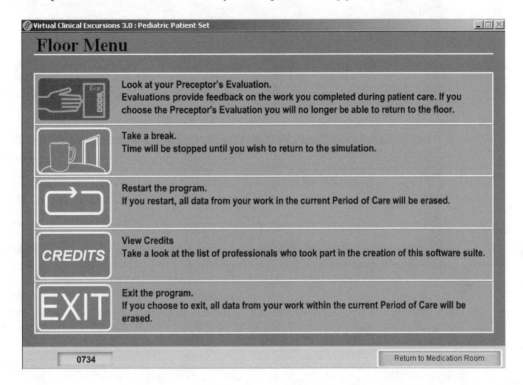

Evaluations are available for each patient you selected when you signed in for the current period of care. Click on the **Medication Scorecard** icon to see an example.

Copyright © 2007 by Saunders, an imprint of Elsevier Inc. All rights reserved.

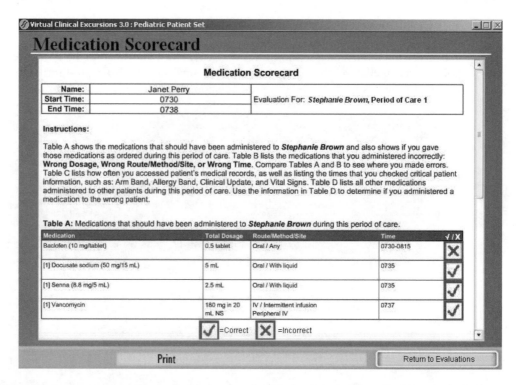

The scorecard compares the medications you administered to a patient during a period of care with what should have been administered. Table A lists the correct medications. Table B lists any medications that were administered incorrectly.

Remember, not every medication listed on the MAR should necessarily be given. For example, a patient might have an allergy to a drug that was ordered, or a medication might have been improperly transcribed to the MAR. Predetermined medication "errors" embedded within the program challenge you to exercise critical thinking skills and professional judgment when deciding to administer a medication, just as you would in a real hospital. Use all your available resources, such as the patient's chart and the MAR, to make your decision.

Table C lists the resources that were available to assist you in medication administration. It also documents whether and when you accessed these resources. For example, did you check the patient armband or perform a check of vital signs? If so, when?

You can click **Print** to get a copy of this report if needed. When you have finished reviewing the scorecard, click **Return to Evaluations** and then **Return to Menu**.

Copyright © 2007 by Saunders, an imprint of Elsevier Inc. All rights reserved.

■ FLOOR MAP

To get a general sense of your location within the hospital, you can click on the **Map** icon found in the lower right corner of most of the screens in the *Virtual Clinical Excursions—Pediatrics* program. (*Note:* If you are following this quick tour step by step, you will need to **Restart the Program** from the Floor Menu, sign in again, and go to the Nurses' Station to access the map.) When you click the **Map** icon, a floor map appears, showing the layout of the floor you are currently on, as well as a directory of the patients and services on that floor. As you move your cursor over the directory list, the location of each room is highlighted on the map (and vice versa). The floor map can be accessed from the Nurses' Station, Medication Room, and each patient's room.

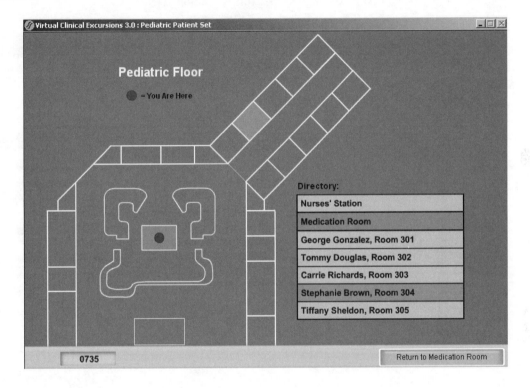

Copyright © 2007 by Saunders, an imprint of Elsevier Inc. All rights reserved.

A DETAILED TOUR

If you wish to more thoroughly understand the capabilities of *Virtual Clinical Excursions—Pediatrics*, take a detailed tour by completing the following section. During this tour, we will work with a specific patient to introduce you to all the different components and learning opportunities available within the software.

■ WORKING WITH A PATIENT

Sign in for Period of Care 1 (0730-0815). From the Patient List, select Stephanie Brown in Room 304; however, do not go to the Nurses' Station yet.

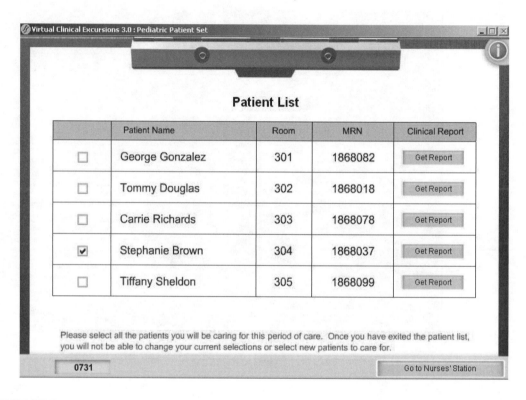

■ REPORT

In hospitals, when one shift ends and another begins, the outgoing nurse who attended a patient will give a verbal and sometimes a written summary of that patient's condition to the incoming nurse who will assume care for the patient. This summary is called a report and is an important source of data to provide an overview of a patient. Your first task is to get the clinical report on Stephanie Brown. To do this, click **Get Report** in the far right column in this patient's row. From a brief review of this summary, identify the problems and areas of concern that you will need to address for this patient.

When you have finished noting any areas of concern, click on **Go to Nurses' Station**.

Copyright © 2007 by Saunders, an imprint of Elsevier Inc. All rights reserved.

■ CHARTS

You can access Stephanie Brown's chart from the Nurses' Station or from the patient's room (304). We will access it from the Nurses' Station: Click on the chart rack or on the **Chart** icon in the tool bar at the top of your screen. Next, click on the chart labeled **304** to open the medical record for Stephanie Brown. Click on the **Emergency Department** tab to view a record of why this patient was admitted.

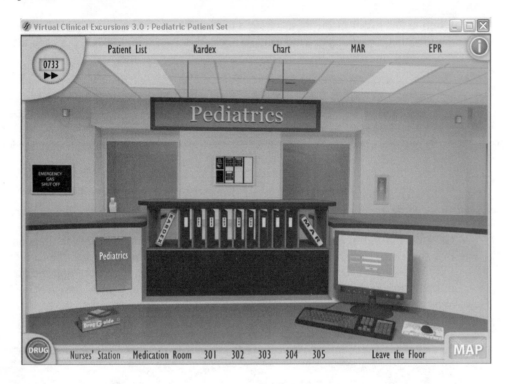

How many days has Stephanie Brown been in the hospital?

What tests were done upon her arrival in the Emergency Department and why?

What was her reason for admission?

You should also click on **Surgical Reports** to learn what procedures were performed and when. Finally, review the **Nursing Admission** and **History and Physical** to learn about the health history of this patient. When you are done reviewing the chart, click **Return to Nurses' Station**.

Copyright © 2007 by Saunders, an imprint of Elsevier Inc. All rights reserved.

■ MEDICATIONS

Open the Medication Administration Record (MAR) by clicking on the **MAR** icon in the tool bar at the top of your screen. *Remember:* The MAR automatically opens to the first occupied room number on the floor—which is not necessarily your patient's room number! Since you need to access Stephanie Brown's MAR, click on tab **304** (her room number). Always make sure you are giving the *Right Drug to the Right Patient!*

Examine the list of medications ordered for Stephanie Brown. In the table below, list the medications that need to be given during this period of care (0730-0815). For each medication, note the dosage, route, and time to be given.

Time	Medication	Dosage	Route

Click on **Return to Nurses' Station**. Next, click on **304** on the bottom tool bar and then verify that you are indeed in Stephanie Brown's room. Select **Clinical Alerts** (the icon to the right of Initial Observations) to check for any emerging data that might affect your medication administration priorities. Next, go to the patient's chart (click on the **Chart** icon; then click on **304**). When the chart opens, select the **Physician's Orders** tab.

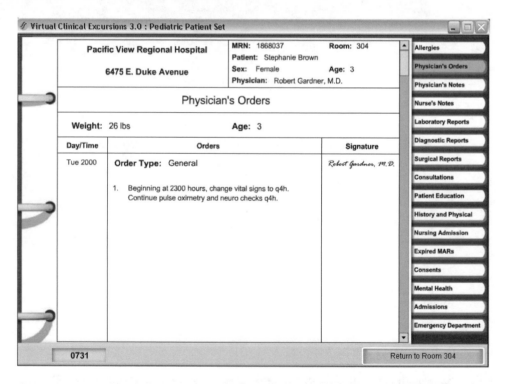

Review the orders. Have any new medications been ordered? Return to the MAR (click **Return to Room 304**; then click **MAR**). Verify that the new medications have been correctly transcribed to the MAR. Mistakes are sometimes made in the transcription process in the hospital setting, and it is sound practice to double-check any new order.

Copyright © 2007 by Saunders, an imprint of Elsevier Inc. All rights reserved.

Are there any patient assessments you will need to perform before administering these medications? If so, return to Room 304 and click on **Patient Care** and then **Physical Assessment** to complete those assessments before proceeding.

Now click on the **Medication Room** icon in the tool bar at the bottom of your screen to locate and prepare the medications for Stephanie Brown.

In the Medication Room, you must access the medications for Stephanie Brown from the specific dispensing system in which each medication is stored. Locate each medication that needs to be given in this time period and click on **Put Medication on Tray** as appropriate. (*Hint:* Look in Unit Dosage drawer first.) When you are finished, click on **Close Drawer** and then on **View Medication Room**. Now click on the medication tray on the counter on the left side of the medication room screen to begin preparing the medications you have selected. (*Remember:* You can also click **Preparation** in the tool bar at top of the screen.)

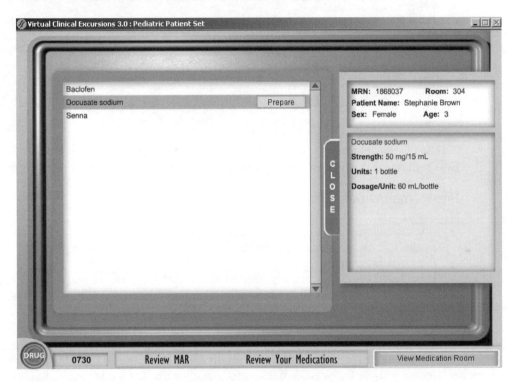

In the preparation area, you should see a list of the medications you put on the tray in the previous steps. Click on the first medication and then click **Prepare**. Follow the onscreen instructions of the Preparation Wizard, providing any data requested. As an example, let's follow the preparation process for docusate sodium, one of the medications due to be administered to Stephanie Brown during this period of care. To begin, click to select **Docusate sodium**; then click **Prepare**. Now work through the Preparation Wizard sequence as detailed below:

> Amount of medication in the bottle: 60 mL.
> Enter the amount of medication you will draw up into a syringe: **5** mL.
> Click **Next**.
> Select the patient you wish to set aside the medication for: **Room 304, Stephanie Brown**.
> Click **Finish**.
> Click **Return to Medication Room**.

Copyright © 2007 by Saunders, an imprint of Elsevier Inc. All rights reserved.

Follow this same basic process for the other medications due to be administered to Stephanie Brown during this period of care. (*Hint:* Look in **IV Storage** and **Automated System**.)

PREPARATION WIZARD EXCEPTIONS

- Some medications in *Virtual Clinical Excursions—Pediatrics* are preprepared by the pharmacy (e.g., IV antibiotics) and taken to the patient room as a whole. This is common practice in most hospitals.
- Blood products are not administered by students through the *Virtual Clinical Excursions— Pediatrics* simulations since blood administration follows specific protocols not covered in this program.
- The *Virtual Clinical Excursions—Pediatrics* simulations do not allow for mixing more than one type of medication, such as regular and Lente insulins, in the same syringe. In the clinical setting, when multiple types of insulin are ordered for a patient, the regular insulin is drawn up first, followed by the longer-acting insulin. Insulin is always administered in a special unit-marked syringe.

Now return to Room 304 (click on **304** on the bottom tool bar) to administer Stephanie Brown's medications.

At any time during the medication administration process, you can perform a further review of systems, take vital signs, check information contained within the chart, or verify patient identity and allergies. Inside Stephanie Brown's room, click **Take Vital Signs**. (*Note:* These findings change over time to reflect the temporal changes you would find in a patient similar to Stephanie Brown.)

Copyright © 2007 by Saunders, an imprint of Elsevier Inc. All rights reserved.

When you have gathered all the data you need, click on **Patient Care** and then select **Medication Administration**. Any medications you prepared in the previous steps should be listed on the left side of your screen. Let's continue the administration process with the vancomycin ordered for Stephanie Brown. Click to highlight **Vancomycin** in the list of medications. Next, click on the down arrow to the right of **Select** and choose **Administer** from the drop-down menu. This will activate the Administration Wizard. Complete the Wizard sequence as follows:

- Route: **IV**
- Method: **Intermittent Infusion**
- Site: **Peripheral IV**
- Click **Administer to Patient** arrow.
- Would you like to document this administration in the MAR? **Yes**
- Click **Finish** arrow.

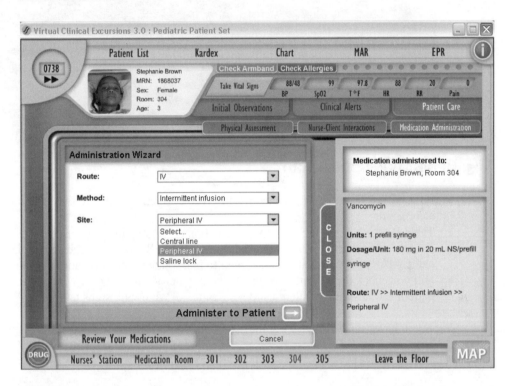

Your selections are recorded by a tracking system and evaluated on a Medication Scorecard stored under Preceptor's Evaluations. This scorecard can be viewed, printed, and given to your instructor. To access the Preceptor's Evaluations, click on **Leave the Floor**. When the Floor Menu appears, click on the icon next to **Look at Your Preceptor's Evaluation**. Then click on **Medication Scorecard** inside the box with Stephanie Brown's name (see example on the following page).

Copyright © 2007 by Saunders, an imprint of Elsevier Inc. All rights reserved.

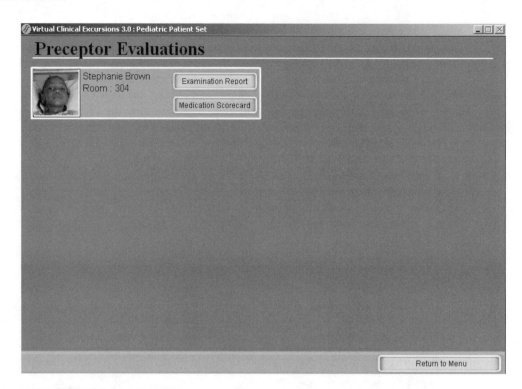

MEDICATION SCORECARD

- First, review Table A. Was vancomycin given correctly? Did you give the other medications as ordered?
- Table B shows you which (if any) medications you gave incorrectly.
- Table C addresses the resources used for Stephanie Brown. Did you access the patient's chart, MAR, EPR, or Kardex as needed to make safe medication administration decisions?
- Did you check the patient's armband to verify her identity? Did you check whether your patient had any known allergies to medications? Were vital signs taken?

When you have finished reviewing the scorecard, click **Return to Evaluations** and then **Return to Menu**.

Copyright © 2007 by Saunders, an imprint of Elsevier Inc. All rights reserved.

■ VITAL SIGNS

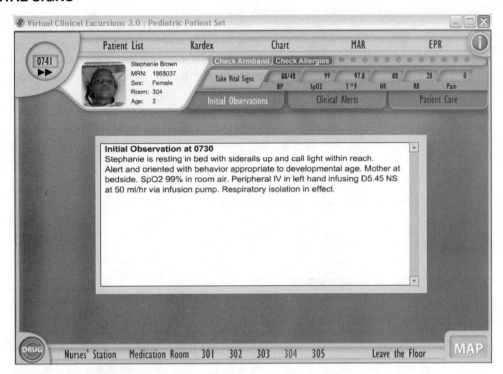

Vital signs, often considered the traditional "signs of life," include body temperature, heart rate, respiratory rate, blood pressure, oxygen saturation of the blood, and pain level.

Inside Stephanie Brown's room, click **Take Vital Signs**. (*Note:* If you are following this detailed tour step by step, you will need to **Restart the Program** from the Floor Menu, sign in again, and navigate to Room 304.) Collect vital signs for this patient and record them in the following table. Note the time at which you collected each of these data. (*Remember:* You can take vital signs at any time. The data change over time to reflect the temporal changes you would find in a patient similar to Stephanie Brown.)

Vital Signs	Findings/Time
Blood pressure	
O$_2$ saturation	
Heart rate	
Respiratory rate	
Temperature	
Pain rating	

Copyright © 2007 by Saunders, an imprint of Elsevier Inc. All rights reserved.

After you are done, click on the **EPR** icon located in the tool bar at the top of the screen. Your username and password are automatically provided. Click on **Login** to enter the EPR. To access Stephanie's records, click on the down arrow next to Patient and choose her room number, **304**. Select **Vital Signs** as the category. Next, in the empty time column on the far right, record the vital signs data you just collected in Stephanie's room. (*Note:* If you need help with this process, see page 16.) Now compare these findings with the data you collected earlier for this patient's vital signs. Use these earlier findings to establish a baseline for each of the vital signs.

a. Are any of the data you collected significantly different from the baseline for a particular vital sign?

Circle One: Yes   No

b. If "Yes," which data are different?

■ PHYSICAL ASSESSMENT

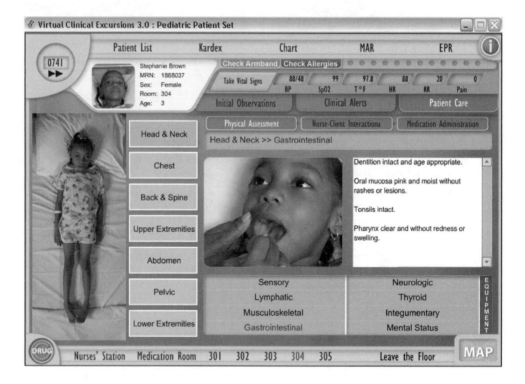

Copyright © 2007 by Saunders, an imprint of Elsevier Inc. All rights reserved.

After you have finished examining the EPR for vital signs, click **Exit EPR** to return to Room 304. Click **Patient Care** and then **Physical Assessment**. Think about what information you received in the report at the beginning of this shift, as well as what you may have learned about this patient from the chart. Based on this, what area(s) of examination should you pay most attention to at this time? Is there any equipment you should be monitoring? Conduct a physical assessment of the body areas and systems that you consider priorities for Stephanie Brown. For example, select **Head & Neck**; then click on and assess **Sensory** and **Lymphatic**. Complete any other assessment(s) you think are necessary at this time. In the following table, record the data you collected during this examination.

Area of Examination	Findings
Head & Neck Sensory	
Head & Neck Lymphatic	

After you have finished collecting these data, return to the EPR. Compare the data that were already in the record with those you just collected.

a. Are any of the data you collected significantly different from the baselines for this patient?

Circle One: Yes   No

b. If "Yes," which data are different?

Copyright © 2007 by Saunders, an imprint of Elsevier Inc. All rights reserved.

■ **NURSE-CLIENT INTERACTIONS**

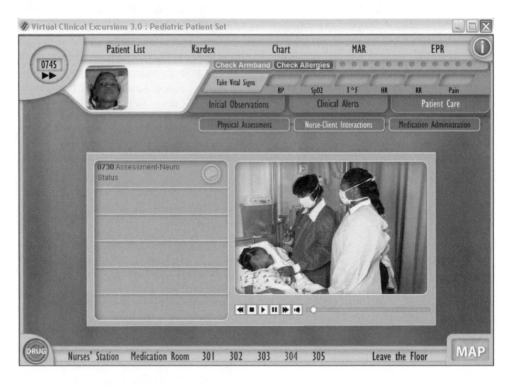

Click on **Patient Care** from inside Stephanie Brown's room (304). Now click on **Nurse-Client Interactions** to access a short video titled **Assessment—Neuro Status**, which is available for viewing at or after 0730 (based on the virtual clock in the upper left corner of your screen; see *Note* below). To begin the video, click on the arrow next to its title. You will observe a nurse explaining her actions to Stephanie's mother. There are many variations of nursing practice, some exemplifying "best" practice and some not. Note whether the nurse in this interaction displays professional behavior and compassionate care. Are her words congruent with what is going on with the patient? Does this interaction "feel right" to you? If not, how would you handle this situation differently? Explain.

Note: If the video you wish to view is not listed, this means you have not yet reached the correct virtual time to view that video. Check the virtual clock; you may return to access the video once its designated time has occurred—as long as you do so within the same period of care. Or you can click on the fast-forward icon within the virtual clock to advance the time by 2-minute intervals. You will then need to click again on **Patient Care** and **Nurse-Client Interactions** to refresh the screen.

At least one Nurse-Client Interactions video is available during each period of care. Viewing these videos can help you learn more about what is occurring with a patient at a certain time and also prompt you to discern between nurse communications that are ideal and those that need improvement. Compassionate care and the ability to communicate clearly are essential components of delivering quality nursing care, and it is during your clinical time that you will begin to refine these skills.

Copyright © 2007 by Saunders, an imprint of Elsevier Inc. All rights reserved.

■ COLLECTING AND EVALUATING DATA

Each of the activities you perform in the Patient Care environment generates a significant amount of assessment data. Remember that after you collect data, you can record your findings in the EPR. You can also review the EPR, patient's chart, videos, and MAR at any time. You will get plenty of practice collecting and then evaluating data in context of the patient's course.

Now, here's an important question for you:

> Did the previous sequence of exercises provide the most efficient way to assess Stephanie Brown?

For example, you went to the patient's room to get vital signs, then back to the EPR to enter data and compare your findings with extant data. Next, you went back to the patient's room to do a physical examination, then again back to the EPR to enter and review data. If this back-and-forth process of data collection and recording seemed inefficient, remember the following:

- Plan all of your nursing activities to maximize efficiency, while at the same time optimizing the quality of patient care. (Think about what data you might need before performing certain tasks. For example, do you need to check a heart rate before administering a cardiac medication or check an IV site before starting an infusion?)

- You collect a tremendous amount of data when you work with a patient. Very few people can accurately remember all these data for more than a few minutes. Develop efficient assessment skills, and record data as soon as possible after collecting them.

- Assessment data are only the starting point for the nursing process.

Make a clear distinction between these first exercises and how you actually provide nursing care. These initial exercises were designed to involve you actively in the use of different software components. This workbook focuses on sensible practices for implementing the nursing process in ways that ensure the highest-quality care of patients.

Most important, remember that a human being changes through time, and that these changes include both the physical and psychosocial facets of a person as a living organism. Think about this for a moment. Some patients may change physically in a very short time (a patient with emerging myocardial infarction) or more slowly (a patient with a chronic illness). Patients' overall physical and psychosocial conditions may improve or deteriorate. They may have effective coping skills and familial support, or they may feel alone and full of despair. In fact, each individual is a complex mix of physical and psychosocial elements, and at least some of these elements usually change through time.

Thus it is crucial that you *DO NOT* think of the nursing process as a simple one-time, five-step procedure consisting of assessment, nursing diagnosis, planning, implementation, and evaluation. Rather, the nursing process should be utilized as a creative and systematic approach to delivering nursing care. Furthermore, because all living organisms are constantly changing, we must apply the nursing process over and over. Each time we follow the nursing process for an individual patient, we refine our understanding of that patient's physical and psychosocial conditions based on collection and analysis of many different types of data. *Virtual Clinical Excursions—Pediatrics* will help you develop both the creativity and the systematic approach needed to become a nurse who is equipped to deliver the highest-quality care to all patients.

Copyright © 2007 by Saunders, an imprint of Elsevier Inc. All rights reserved.

REDUCING MEDICATION ERRORS

Earlier in this detailed tour, you learned the basic steps of medication preparation and administration. The following simulations will allow you to practice those skills further—with an increased emphasis on reducing medication errors by using the Medication Scorecard to evaluate your work.

Sign in to work at Pacific View Regional Hospital for Period of Care 1. (*Note:* If you are already working with another patient or during another period of care, click on **Leave the Floor** and then **Restart the Program**; then sign in.)

From the Patient List, select Stephanie Brown. Then click on **Go to Nurses' Station**. Complete the following steps to prepare and administer medications to Stephanie Brown.

- Click on **Medication Room**.
- Click on **MAR** and then on tab **304** to determine prn medications that have been ordered for Stephanie Brown to address her constipation and pain. (*Note:* You may click on **Review MAR** at any time to verify the correct medication order. Always remember to check the patient name on the MAR to make sure you have the correct patient's record—you must click on the correct room number tab within the MAR.) Click on **Return to Medication Room** after reviewing the correct MAR.
- Click on **Unit Dosage** (or on the Unit Dosage cabinet); from the close-up view, click on drawer **304**.
- Select the medications you would like to administer. After each selection, click **Put Medication on Tray**. When you are finished selecting medications, click **Close Drawer** and then **View Medication Room**.
- Click on **Automated System** (or on the Automated System unit itself). Click **Login**.
- On the next screen, specify the correct patient and drawer location.
- Select the medication you would like to administer and click on **Put Medication on Tray**. Repeat this process if you wish to administer other medications from the Automated System.
- When you are finished, click **Close Drawer** and **View Medication Room**.
- From the Medication Room, click on **Preparation** (or on the preparation tray).
- From the list of medications on your tray, highlight the correct medication to administer and click **Prepare**.
- This activates the Preparation Wizard. Supply any requested information; then click **Next**.
- Now select the correct patient to receive this medication and click **Finish**.
- Repeat the previous three steps until all medications that you want to administer are prepared.
- You can click on **Review Your Medications** and then on **Return to Medication Room** when ready. Once you are back in the Medication Room, go directly to Stephanie Brown's room by clicking on **304** at bottom of screen.
- Inside the patient's room, administer the medication, utilizing the five rights of medication administration. After you have collected the appropriate assessment data and are ready for administration, click **Patient Care** and then **Medication Administration**. Verify that the correct patient and medication(s) appear in the left-hand window. Highlight the first medication you wish to administer; then click the down arrow next to Select. From the drop-down menu, select **Administer** and complete the Administration Wizard by providing any information requested. When the Wizard stops asking for information, click **Administer to Patient**. Specify **Yes** when asked whether this administration should be recorded in the MAR. Finally, click **Finish**.

Copyright © 2007 by Saunders, an imprint of Elsevier Inc. All rights reserved.

■ SELF-EVALUATION

Now let's see how you did during your medication administration!

- Click on **Leave the Floor** at the bottom of your screen. From the Floor Menu, select **Look at Your Preceptor's Evaluation**. Then click on **Medication Scorecard** for Stephanie Brown. These resources will help you find out more about each patient's medications and possible sources of medication errors.

1. Start by examining Table A. These are the medications you should have given to Stephanie Brown during this period of care. If each of the medications in Table A has a ✓ by it, then you made no errors. Congratulations!

If any medication has an X by it, then you made one or more medication errors.

Compare Tables A and B to determine which of the following types of errors you made: Wrong Dose, Wrong Route/Method/Site, or Wrong Time. Follow these steps:
   a. Find medications in Table A that were given incorrectly.
   b. Now see if those same medications are in Table B, which shows what you actually administered to Stephanie Brown.
   c. Comparing Tables A and B, match the Strength, Dose, Route/Method/Site, and Time for each medication you administered incorrectly.
   d. Then, using the form below, list the medications given incorrectly and mark the errors you made for each medication.

Medication	Strength	Dosage	Route	Method	Site	Time
	❑	❑	❑	❑	❑	❑
	❑	❑	❑	❑	❑	❑
	❑	❑	❑	❑	❑	❑
	❑	❑	❑	❑	❑	❑

2. To help you reduce future medication errors, consider the following list of possible reasons for errors.

   - Did not check drug against MAR for correct patient, correct date, correct time, correct drug, and correct dose.
   - Did not check drug dose against MAR three times.
   - Did not open the unit dose package in the patient's room.
   - Did not correctly identify the patient using two identifiers.
   - Did not administer the drug on time.
   - Did not verify patient allergies.
   - Did not check the patient's current condition or vital sign parameters.
   - Did not consider why the patient would be receiving this drug.
   - Did not question why the drug was in the patient's drawer.
   - Did not check the physician's order and/or check with the pharmacist when there was a question about the drug or dose.
   - Did not verify that no adverse effects had occurred from a previous dose.

Copyright © 2007 by Saunders, an imprint of Elsevier Inc. All rights reserved.

Based on these possibilities, determine how you made each error and record the reason in the form below:

Medication	Reason for Error

3. Look again at Table B. Are there medications listed that are not in Table A? If so, you gave a medication to Stephanie Brown that she should not have received. Complete the following exercises to help you understand how such an error might have been made.

   a. Perhaps you gave a medication that was on Stephanie Brown's MAR for this period of care, without recognizing that a change had occurred in the patient's condition, which should have caused you to reconsider. Review patient records as necessary and complete the following form:

Medication	Possible Reasons Not to Give This Medication

   b. Another possibility is that you gave Stephanie Brown a medication that should have been given at a different time. Check her MAR and complete the form below to determine whether you made a Wrong Time error:

Medication	Given to Stephanie Brown at What Time	Should Have Been Given at What Time

Copyright © 2007 by Saunders, an imprint of Elsevier Inc. All rights reserved.

c. Maybe you gave another patient's medication to Stephanie Brown. In this case, you made a Wrong Patient error. Check the MARs of other patients and use the form below to determine whether you made this type of error:

Medication	Given to Stephanie Brown	Should Have Been Given to

4. The Medication Scorecard provides some other interesting sources of information. For example, if there is a medication selected for Stephanie Brown but it was not given to her, there will be an X by that medication in Table A, but it will not appear in Table B. In that case, you might have given this medication to some other patient, which is another type of Wrong Patient error. To investigate further, look at Table D, which lists the medications you gave to other patients. See whether you can find any medications for Stephanie Brown that were given to another patient by mistake. However, before you make any decisions, be sure to cross-check the MAR for other patients because the same medication may have been ordered for multiple patients. Use the following form to record your findings:

Medication	Should Have Been Given to Stephanie Brown	Given by Mistake to

Copyright © 2007 by Saunders, an imprint of Elsevier Inc. All rights reserved.

5. Now take some time to review the medication exercises you just completed. Use the form below to create an overall analysis of what you have learned. Once again, record each of the medication errors you made, including the type of each error. Then, for each error you made, indicate specifically what you would do differently to prevent this type of error from occurring again.

Medication	Type of Error	Error Prevention Tactic

Submit this form to your instructor if required as a graded assignment, or simply use these exercises to improve your understanding of medication errors and how to reduce them.

Name: _____   Date: _____

Copyright © 2007 by Saunders, an imprint of Elsevier Inc. All rights reserved.

The following icons are used throughout the workbook to help you quickly identify particular activities and assignments:

 Indicates a reading assignment—tells you which textbook chapter(s) you should read before starting each lesson

 Indicates a writing activity

 Marks the beginning of an interactive CD-ROM activity—signals you to open or return to your *Virtual Clinical Excursions—Pediatrics* CD-ROM

 Indicates additional CD-ROM instructions

 Indicates questions and activities that require you to consult your textbook

 Indicates the approximate time required to complete an exercise

Copyright © 2007 by Saunders, an imprint of Elsevier Inc. All rights reserved.

LESSON **1** _____

The Hospitalized Infant

_____

👓 **Reading Assignment:** Health Promotion for the Developing Child
(Chapter 4, pages 64-72, 80-83, 86-90)
Health Promotion for the Infant (Chapter 5, pages 98-132)
The Ill Child in the Hospital and Other Care Settings
(Chapter 11, pages 288-290)

Patient: Carrie Richards, Room 303

Objectives:

- Identify developmental milestones for the first year of life.
- Score a DDST II on an infant and discuss the implications of this score.
- Discuss the needs of the hospitalized infant.
- Determine nursing interventions necessary for promoting growth and development of the hospitalized infant.
- Determine the immunization needs of the infant.
- Identify areas for anticipatory guidance for a selected hospitalized infant.
- Discuss parental needs while an infant is hospitalized.

In this lesson you will be caring for a hospitalized infant whose mother stays with her most of the time. You will learn how to consider growth and development when planning and implementing care. You will learn how to promote development in the hospitalized infant. Additionally, you will learn how to anticipate and be responsive to parental needs.

Copyright © 2007 by Saunders, an imprint of Elsevier Inc. All rights reserved.

Exercise 1

 CD-ROM Activity

 45 minutes

1. For each category of growth and development listed in the chart below, provide an example of an accomplishment for an infant that would be observable by parents at each age.

Area	2 Months	4 Months	6 Months	12 Months
Physical growth				
Motor skills				
Psychosocial development				
Sensory and cognitive development				
Language and communication skills				

Copyright © 2007 by Saunders, an imprint of Elsevier Inc. All rights reserved.

2. Did you include social smiling in question 1? If so, to which area and age did you assign this behavior?

3. At what point should the nurse be concerned when a growth and development milestone and/or behavior is not observed?

 • Sign in to work at Pacific View Regional Hospital for Period of Care 1. (*Note:* If you are already in the virtual hospital from a previous exercise, click on **Leave the Floor** and then **Restart the Program** to get to the sign-in window.)

• From the Patient List, select Carrie Richards (Room 303).

• Click on **Go to Nurses' Station**.

• Click on **Chart** and then on **303**.

• Click on **History and Physical** and review this section.

4. In the table below, list the information you found in Carrie Richards' History and Physical related to her growth and development. You are being asked to recognize the significance of information, as well as to consider the factors that have affected—or may affect—growth and development. Show connections or relationships you see by providing rationales as to why the factor you cited has an influence. An example has been provided.

Assessment Data	Contributing Factors	Rationales
Small and thin for age	Mother is a smoker.	Creates an unhealthy environment

Copyright © 2007 by Saunders, an imprint of Elsevier Inc. All rights reserved.

5. What is Erikson's developmental task for infancy? Generally, what needs to happen in order for development to occur in this area?

6. How can the above task be promoted in the hospital situation?

7. What does Piaget say about this stage of development?

8. Consider Piaget's theory as you reflect on infant behavior. Are there any safety implications?

9. Identify areas related to growth and development that you would like to assess in Carrie Richards while she is hospitalized.

Copyright © 2007 by Saunders, an imprint of Elsevier Inc. All rights reserved.

10. Give an example of age-appropriate play for Carrie Richards and identify what developmental needs are being met through this type of play.

Exercise 2

 CD-ROM Activity

 30 minutes

- Sign in to work at Pacific View Regional Hospital for Period of Care 1. (*Note:* If you are already in the virtual hospital from a previous exercise, click on **Leave the Floor** and then **Restart the Program** to get to the sign-in window.)
- From the Patient List, select Carrie Richards (Room 303).
- Click on **Get Report** and review the clinical report.
- Click on **Go to Nurses' Station**.
- Click on **Chart** and then on **303**.
- Click on and review the **History and Physical**, **Nursing Admission**, and **Emergency Department** sections of the chart.

 1. Review the information on the DDST II in your textbook. (*Hint:* See pages 80-83.) Using the DDST II chart found on your textbook's Evolve website, plot the information you have about Carrie Richards. Below, list the behaviors that she should have accomplished completely by now. What are some that she may have achieved (over the 50% mark)?

Copyright © 2007 by Saunders, an imprint of Elsevier Inc. All rights reserved.

• Click on **Return to Nurses' Station** and then on **303**.
• Click on **Patient Care** and then on **Physical Assessment**.
• Perform a complete physical assessment, paying particular attention to data that are relevant to the DDST II.

2. Note your assessment findings below.

3. The DDST II is a screening test. Explain how such a test is used.

4. How would you, in your own words, explain the test to Carrie Richards' mother?

5. Discuss whether or not it is appropriate to perform the Denver Developmental Screening Test on infants and children in the hospital.

Copyright © 2007 by Saunders, an imprint of Elsevier Inc. All rights reserved.

Exercise 3

 CD-ROM Activity

 30 minutes

- Sign in to work at Pacific View Regional Hospital for Period of Care 1. (*Note:* If you are already in the virtual hospital from a previous exercise, click on **Leave the Floor** and then **Restart the Program** to get to the sign-in window.)
- From the Patient List, select Carrie Richards (Room 303).
- Click on **Go to Nurses' Station** and then on **303**.
- Click on **Patient Care** and then on **Nurse-Client Interactions**.
- Select and view the video titled **0730: Patient Assessment**. (*Note:* Check the virtual clock to see whether enough time has elapsed. You can use the fast-forward feature to advance the time by 2-minute intervals if the video is not yet available. Then click again on **Patient Care** and **Nurse-Client Interactions** to refresh the screen.)

1. What positive parenting behaviors do you observe in this interaction between Carrie Richards and her mother that promote the meeting of developmental tasks?

 - Click on **Chart** and then on **303**.
- Click on the **History and Physical** tab and review this section.

2. Check Carrie Richards' record for her immunization status. What teaching is indicated?

3. What immunizations does Carrie Richards now need?

Copyright © 2007 by Saunders, an imprint of Elsevier Inc. All rights reserved.

4. List two or three areas of anticipatory guidance related to growth and development and health promotion that you could discuss with Carrie Richards' mother.

5. Considering your response to the previous question, discuss the appropriate methods for helping Carrie Richards' mother learn.

6. Consider what might happen if Carrie Richards' hospital stay is extended and her mother says that she can't leave because she is afraid Carrie will cry. What would you say to her in your own words?

7. Consider now an opposite situation in which Carrie Richards' mother does not spend much time at the hospital. Discuss your thoughts and how you would address the situation.

Great job! You are now ready to take this growth and development knowledge and apply it as you consider further the care of an ill infant.

Copyright © 2007 by Saunders, an imprint of Elsevier Inc. All rights reserved.

LESSON 2

Caring for an Infant with Bronchiolitis

⌒○⌒ **Reading Assignment:** Health Promotion for the Infant (Chapter 5, pages 98-132)

Principles and Procedures for Nursing Care of Children
(Chapter 13, pages 336-338, 341-346, 353, 360-361)

The Child with a Respiratory Alteration
(Chapter 21, pages 601, 623-626)

Patient: Carrie Richards, Room 303

Objectives:

- Discuss the etiology and pathophysiology of bronchiolitis.
- Explain the relationship between infant growth and bronchiolitis.
- Complete a respiratory assessment on an infant and discuss nursing care issues.
- Use the nursing process to develop a nursing care plan for an infant with bronchiolitis and the family.

In this lesson you will learn and reinforce concepts related to a common respiratory illness in infants, bronchiolitis. You will apply principles of growth and development in making nursing care decisions. You will be expected to recall/review basic oral and written communication, teaching skills, and family-centered care. Your patient is Carrie Richards, a 3½-month-old who has been admitted to the Pediatric Unit from the Emergency Department. Carrie's medical diagnosis is bronchiolitis. Her mother is with her.

Copyright © 2007 by Saunders, an imprint of Elsevier Inc. All rights reserved.

Exercise 1

 Clinical Preparation: Writing Activity

 15 minutes

1. Explain the pathophysiology of bronchiolitis.

2. Identify the most common etiologic agent associated with bronchiolitis and explain its relationship to bronchiolitis.

3. Discuss infant growth and development as it relates to physiologic function of the respiratory system.

Copyright © 2007 by Saunders, an imprint of Elsevier Inc. All rights reserved.

4. Think about how you would explain a diagnosis of bronchiolitis to Carrie Richards' mother. What information would you share? How would you present it?

Exercise 2

  CD-ROM Activity

30 minutes

- Sign in to work at Pacific View Regional Hospital for Period of Care 1. (*Note:* If you are already in the virtual hospital from a previous exercise, click on **Leave the Floor** and then **Restart the Program** to get to the sign-in window.)
- From the Patient List, select Carrie Richards (Room 303).
- Click on **Go to Nurses' Station**.
- Click on **Chart** and then on **303**.
- Click on and review the **History and Physical**, **Nursing Admission**, and **Emergency Department** tabs.

1. As you read these records, list the data that are consistent with bronchiolitis.

Copyright © 2007 by Saunders, an imprint of Elsevier Inc. All rights reserved.

2. What do these observations indicate regarding Carrie Richards' health status? How do you interpret the seriousness of her illness? Do you think she is mildly or seriously ill? Explain your response.

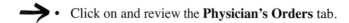 • Click on and review the **Physician's Orders** tab.

3. What is the rationale for the physician's orders for IV fluids, medications, oxygen, pulse oximetry, and lab work? (*Hint:* To review medication information, click on the Drug icon in the lower left corner of your screen. You can review the Drug Guide from either the Nurses' Station or the patient's room. You may also refer to a nursing drug handbook if you need more information.)

4. Carrie Richards had nasal washing performed while she was in the ED. What is nasal washing, and what are the nursing responsibilities for carrying out this procedure?

Copyright © 2007 by Saunders, an imprint of Elsevier Inc. All rights reserved.

5. If you were performing the nasal washing procedure on Carrie Richards, would you anticipate needing to restrain her? If so, what type of restraint would you use? Would you ask Carrie's mother to help? (*Hint:* Check Carrie's physical status and behavior while in the ED.)

6. Explain the type of isolation being used. (*Hint:* Check the Physician's Orders in the chart. You may also want to review the information in the Standard Precautions section on the textbook's Evolve website.)

Copyright © 2007 by Saunders, an imprint of Elsevier Inc. All rights reserved.

7. What other infection-control precautions should be implemented?

8. Define *nosocomial infection*.

9. Why must care be taken to prevent Carrie Richards from developing a nosocomial infection?

→ • Click on **Return to Nurses' Station** and then on **303** at the bottom of the screen.
  • Click on **Patient Care**.
  • Click on **Nurse-Client Interactions**.
  • Select and view the video titled **0730: Patient Assessment**. (*Note:* Check the virtual clock to see whether enough time has elapsed. You can use the fast-forward feature to advance the time by 2-minute intervals if the video is not yet available. Then click again on **Patient Care** and **Nurse-Client Interactions** to refresh the screen.)

10. What actions, if any, by the mother or the nurse are inappropriate in this interaction?

Copyright © 2007 by Saunders, an imprint of Elsevier Inc. All rights reserved.

Exercise 3

  CD-ROM Activity

45 minutes

- Sign in to work at Pacific View Regional Hospital for Period of Care 1. (*Note:* If you are already in the virtual hospital from a previous exercise, click on **Leave the Floor** and then **Restart the Program** to get to the sign-in window.)
- From the Patient List, select Carrie Richards (Room 303).
- Click on **Go to Nurses' Station** and the on **303**.
- Inside the patient's room, click on **Check Armband** and then on **Take Vital Signs**.
- Next, click on **Patient Care** and complete a head-to-toe physical assessment by clicking on the various categories and subcategories.

1. What are Carrie Richards' vital signs? Are they within normal limits? Are you concerned about any of these findings?

2. Based on your assessment, list any observations that reflect Carrie's oxygenation status.

3. Which method would you use to take Carrie's temperature?
   a. Axillary
   b. Oral
   c. Rectal
   d. Tympanic

4. When using this type of thermometer, how should the pinna of Carrie's ear be positioned?
   a. Down and back
   b. Up and forward
   c. Up and back
   d. Straight back

Copyright © 2007 by Saunders, an imprint of Elsevier Inc. All rights reserved.

5. Carrie Richards is of African-American descent. What is the best way to assess color in a dark-skinned person?

 • Click on **EPR** and then on **Login**.
- Select **303** as the Patient and **Vital Signs** as the Category. Use the blue backward and forward arrows as needed to document these data your assessment findings in the appropriate time columns.
- Continue to chart your observations in the **Respiratory** and **Cardiovascular** categories.

6. If you missed anything, go back to Carrie Richards' room and reassess her. Because the EPR format is generic, you may not have data for all areas listed. You do, however, need to make sure you are recognizing significant assessment data. Review data trends since her admission. What is your assessment of Carrie's status? Why is continued monitoring necessary?

 • Click on **Exit EPR** to return to Carrie Richards' room.
- Click on **Patient Care**.
- Based on your previous findings and your answer to question 6, perform a focused assessment of Carrie.
- Click on **Leave the Floor** and then on **Look at Your Preceptor's Evaluations**.
- Click on and review the **Examination Report**. You may print the Examination Report if you wish.

7. How did you do with your focused assessment? Do you note any gaps? Were you efficient and systemic? Is there any area for improvement in your performance?

 • Click on **Return to Evaluations**.
- Click on **Return to Menu** and then **Restart the Program**.
- Sign in to work at Pacific View Regional Hospital for Period of Care 1.
- From the Patient List, select Carrie Richards (Room 303).
- Click on **Go to Nurses' Station**.
- Click on **EPR** and then **Login**.
- Select Carrie Richards' EPR (**303**) and document your latest assessment findings.

Copyright © 2007 by Saunders, an imprint of Elsevier Inc. All rights reserved.

8. Is Carrie's condition improving or deteriorating?

9. Consider the possibility of Carrie Richards' condition deteriorating. What changes might you anticipate that would indicate worsening of her health status?

10. How is Carrie receiving oxygen?

11. Sometimes oxygen is delivered in a mist tent. What are the nursing responsibilities for care of an infant in a mist tent? Are there any advantages to using a mist tent rather than a nasal cannula?

Copyright © 2007 by Saunders, an imprint of Elsevier Inc. All rights reserved.

12. How is Carrie Richards' O_2 status being monitored? What should the nurse be looking for?

13. Documentation is important. What information is necessary for documenting observations associated with Carrie's O_2 saturation levels?

14. Oxygenation assessment is ongoing. In older children and adults, the nurse can easily assess respiratory status in response to play or other activity. How can this ongoing assessment be carried out in an infant?

Exercise 4

 Clinical Preparation: Writing Activity

 30 minutes

1. You have completed an oxygenation assessment. Write the priority nursing diagnosis for Carrie Richards at this time. (*Hint:* You may find it useful to check distinguishing characteristics for the various oxygenation nursing diagnoses in a nursing diagnosis book.)

Copyright © 2007 by Saunders, an imprint of Elsevier Inc. All rights reserved.

2. List below the goals with outcomes for your priority nursing diagnosis. You may write these in the format required by your nursing program.

3. Develop nursing interventions for the nursing diagnosis you identified above. Make sure you include time frames and amounts where appropriate.

4. Evaluate your goals. Create an evaluation statement that reflects achievement of goals. (*Hint:* Specific outcomes need to be included here.)

Copyright © 2007 by Saunders, an imprint of Elsevier Inc. All rights reserved.

5. Now create an evaluation statement that reflects goals that are not met.

Congratulations! You have completed a comprehensive review of bronchiolitis and several aspects of nursing care. Proceed to Lesson 3 to learn about other specific challenges in the care of an infant with a respiratory illness.

Copyright © 2007 by Saunders, an imprint of Elsevier Inc. All rights reserved.

Nursing Care Issues Associated with Bronchiolitis

Reading Assignment: Medicating Infants and Children
(Chapter 14, pages 372-379, 386-391)
The Child with a Fluid and Electrolyte Alteration
(Chapter 18, pages 487-498)
The Child with a Respiratory Alteration
(Chapter 21, pages 623-626)

Patient: Carrie Richards, Room 303

Objectives:

- Discuss the reasons that infants are at risk for hydration problems.
- Explain the risk for dehydration in infants with respiratory illnesses.
- Discuss nursing care for managing hydration concerns, including IV therapy.
- Practice oral medication administration in infants.
- Identify and discuss areas for independent teaching in the care of infants.
- Discuss discharge teaching responsibilities for the patient with bronchiolitis.

In this lesson you will explore hydration as an area of concern in infants with respiratory problems. You will also explore oral medication administration and practice it in a virtual sense. You will consider the role of the nurse related to a variety of teaching areas: the illness and discharge teaching, medication administration, and growth and development. You will need to recall and use the principles of good communication and teaching-learning as you continue to work with Carrie Richards and her mother.

Copyright © 2007 by Saunders, an imprint of Elsevier Inc. All rights reserved.

Exercise 1

 CD-ROM Activity

 60 minutes

1. List the characteristics of infants that put them at greater risk for hydration problems. Underline those that particularly relate to dehydration as a potential problem with respiratory illness.

2. List the areas you would want to assess in completing a hydration assessment in an infant.

Copyright © 2007 by Saunders, an imprint of Elsevier Inc. All rights reserved.

• Sign in to work at Pacific View Regional Hospital for Period of Care 1. (*Note:* If you are already in the virtual hospital from a previous exercise, click on **Leave the Floor** and then **Restart the Program** to get to the sign-in window.)

• From the Patient List, select Carrie Richards (Room 303).

• Click on **Get Report** and read the clinical report.

• Click on **Go to Nurses' Station** and then on **303**.

• Click on **Patient Care** and complete a focused assessment of Carrie Richards. (*Remember:* A focused assessment is one that reflects the priority health concern as well as those concerns for which the patient is at risk.)

• Once your assessment is complete, click on **EPR** and then **Login**.

• Select **303** as the Patient and choose categories as needed to record the data from your focused assessment. (*Hint:* If you need help entering data in the EPR, refer to pages 15-16 in the **Getting Started** section of this workbook.)

• When you have finished documenting your assessments, click on **Exit EPR**.

• Now, to see how you did, click on **Leave the Floor**.

• From the Floor Menu, select **Look at Your Preceptor's Evaluations**.

• Now click on **Examination Report** and review the feedback.

3. Reflect on your performance with this assessment. Did you assess both respiratory status and hydration? Remember that each affects the other.

4. What important hydration assessment parameters can you use with Carrie Richards that would not be available with an older child?

5. What is the most reliable information you can use to assess an infant's hydration status? Why?

6. Identify the guidelines for obtaining daily weights in a manner that will provide meaningful information.

Now let's jump ahead in virtual time to practice your focused assessment again.

 • Click on **Return to Evaluations**, then on **Return to Menu**, and finally **Restart the Program**.

• Sign in to work at Pacific View Regional Hospital for Period of Care 2.

• From the Patient List, select Carrie Richards (Room 303).

• Click on **Go to Nurses' Station** and then on **303**.

• Complete a focused assessment and chart your findings in the EPR.

• When you have finished documenting your assessments, click on **Exit EPR**.

• Now, to see how you did, click on **Leave the Floor**.

• From the Floor Menu, select **Look at Your Preceptor's Evaluations**.

• Now click on **Examination Report** and review the feedback.

7. Reflect on how you are doing with your focused assessments. Consider completeness, comfort, efficiency, and skill. Are you feeling more confident about your thoroughness?

Now practice your focused assessment once more, this time in Period of Care 3.

 • Click on **Return to Evaluations**, then on **Return to Menu**, and finally **Restart the Program**.

• Sign in to work at Pacific View Regional Hospital for Period of Care 3.

• From the Patient List, select Carrie Richards (Room 303).

• Click on **Go to Nurses' Station** and then on **303**.

• Complete a focused assessment and chart your findings in the EPR.

• When you have finished documenting your assessments, click on **Exit EPR**.

• Now, to see how you did, click on **Leave the Floor**.

• From the Floor Menu, select **Look at Your Preceptor's Evaluations**.

• Now click on **Examination Report** and review the feedback.

Copyright © 2007 by Saunders, an imprint of Elsevier Inc. All rights reserved.

8. Once more, reflect on how you are doing with your focused assessment. What improvements have you made? What have you learned? Is there still room for more improvement?

 • Click on **Return to Evaluations**, then on **Return to Menu**, and finally **Restart the Program**.
   • Sign in to work at Pacific View Regional Hospital for Period of Care 1.
   • From the Patient List, select Carrie Richards (Room 303).
   • Click on **Go to Nurses' Station** and then on **303**.
   • Click on **Patient Care** and then on **Nurse-Client Interactions**.
   • Select and view the video titled **0730: Patient Assessment**. (*Note:* Check the virtual clock to see whether enough time has elapsed. You can use the fast-forward feature to advance the time by 2-minute intervals if the video is not yet available. Then click again on **Patient Care** and **Nurse-Client Interactions** to refresh the screen.)

9. Evaluate the nurse's assessment of the IV site. What should the nurse be looking for? Was she thorough in her assessment?

10. Discuss the nursing responsibilities associated with IV fluid administration in infants. (*Hint:* Remember that IV fluid is considered a medication.)

Copyright © 2007 by Saunders, an imprint of Elsevier Inc. All rights reserved.

11. What factors determine site selection for the IV insertion?

12. What is unique about scalp veins? Why are they frequently used in infants?

13. You find that infusion pumps are in very short supply. You know that Carrie Richards, because of her age, needs a pump and that she will get the next available one. In the meantime, you must anticipate using IV tubing that has a burette. What is the rationale for use of this type of tubing?

→ • Click on **Chart** and then on **303**.
   • Click on and review the **Nursing Admission** tab.

14. Calculate Carrie Richards' daily fluid maintenance needs. Determine minimum urine output. (*Hint:* You will need to find her weight in the Nursing Admission form to make this calculation.)

15. What would you tell Carrie Richards' mother about adequate hydration? How will she know whether her baby is getting enough fluids?

Copyright © 2007 by Saunders, an imprint of Elsevier Inc. All rights reserved.

→ • Now click on the **Physician's Orders** tab and find the most recent order for IV fluids for Carrie Richards.

16. Carrie Richards is receiving an IV infusion with potassium added. Verify the order by checking the Physician's Orders. Explain what she is receiving. Discuss the nurse's responsibilities related to potassium administration to an infant.

17. Consider what aspects of care (with regard to managing the IV) you may assign to Carrie Richards' mother. What could you ask her to do while still maintaining safe care and fulfilling your legal responsibility?

18. Explain what is meant by *oral rehydration therapy (ORT)*.

Copyright © 2007 by Saunders, an imprint of Elsevier Inc. All rights reserved.

Exercise 2

 CD-ROM Activity

 30 minutes

- Sign in to work at Pacific View Regional Hospital Period of Care 3. (*Note:* If you are already in the virtual hospital from a previous exercise, click on **Leave the Floor** and then **Restart the Program** to get to the sign-in window.)
- From the Patient List, select Carrie Richards (Room 303).
- Click on **Go to Nurses' Station** and then on **303**.
- Click on **Take Vital Signs**.
- Click on **Clinical Alerts** and review the report.

1. Can Carrie Richards have Tylenol? If so, for what reason will you be giving it?

2. What should you check before you prepare the medication? (*Hint:* Consider the specific need for this medication, as well as the nursing responsibilities before administering any medication.)

→ • Click on **MAR** and find the order for this medication.

3. Is the ordered dose of this medication appropriate for Carrie Richards? If not, why not?

Copyright © 2007 by Saunders, an imprint of Elsevier Inc. All rights reserved.

4. Assume that Carrie Richards had an order for an antibiotic that read "40 mg/kg/day PO in divided doses every 8 hours." How much would you give for each dose?

5. What are the appropriate methods for administering oral medications to an infant?

- Click on **Return to Room 303**.
- Click on **Medication Room** and then **Unit Dosage**.
- Click on **Drawer 303**.
- Click on **Acetaminophen** and then **Put Medication on Tray**.
- Click on **Close Drawer**.
- Click on **View Medication Room**.
- Click on **Preparation** and then **Prepare**. Follow the Preparation Wizard's prompts to complete preparation of Carrie Richards' acetaminophen dose.
- Click on **Return to Medication Room**.
- Click on **303** to return to Carrie Richards' room.
- Click on **Check Armband**.
- Click on **Check Allergies**.
- Click on **Patient Care** and then **Medication Administration**.
- Find **Acetaminophen** listed on the left side of your screen. Click on the down arrow next to Select and choose **Administer**.
- Follow the Administration Wizard's prompts to administer the medication. Indicate Yes to document the administration in the MAR.
- Click on **Leave the Floor**.
- Click on **Look at Your Preceptor's Evaluations**.
- Click on **Medication Scorecard**. How did you do?

6. Did you get check marks indicating that you completed the medication administration procedure satisfactorily? What, if anything, did you forget? What, if anything, would you do differently?

Copyright © 2007 by Saunders, an imprint of Elsevier Inc. All rights reserved.

You have just been walked through the medication preparation and administration procedure. Now try it on your own. To do so, you have two options:

 • Click on **MAR** and see whether Carrie Richards has any other medications due at this time. If she does, you can stay in this period of care and proceed with the preparation and administration.

• If you prefer to practice preparing and giving Carrie Richards the same acetaminophen dose you just completed, click on **Leave the Floor** and then **Restart the Program**. Sign in again to work with Carrie Richards for Period of Care 3 and proceed from there.

Regardless of which option you choose, remember to follow the Six Rights! After you have finished administering the medication, be sure to see how you did by checking your Medication Scorecard.

• Click on **Leave the Floor** and then on **Look at Your Preceptor's Evaluations**.
• Click on **Medication Scorecard** and review your evaluation.

Now let's jump back in virtual time to visit Carrie Richards earlier in the day.

• First, click on **Return to Evaluations**, then on **Return to Menu**, and then on **Restart the Program**.
• Sign in to work at Pacific View Regional Hospital for Period of Care 2.
• From the Patient List, select Carrie Richards (Room 303).
• Click on **Go to Nurses' Station** and then on **303**.
• Click on **Patient Care** and then on **Nurse-Client Interactions**.
• Select and view the video titled **1115: Nutritional Assessment**. The focus of this interaction is on application of teaching-learning principles rather than nutritional assessment. (*Note:* Check the virtual clock to see whether enough time has elapsed. You can use the fast-forward feature to advance the time by 2-minute intervals if the video is not yet available. Then click again on **Patient Care** and **Nurse-Client Interactions** to refresh the screen.)

7. Share your thoughts on the nurse's teaching. Consider the teaching-learning principles that are depicted.

Copyright © 2007 by Saunders, an imprint of Elsevier Inc. All rights reserved.

8. Carrie Richards' mother needs to know how to give Carrie her medication at home. How will you determine whether she is skillful and comfortable enough giving her baby medication?

9. How would you respond to the following concern: "The nurse is supposed to give the medication, so how can the nurse allow a parent to administer medication?" (*Hint:* To answer this, you need to think through the nurse's legal responsibilities.)

Exercise 3

 Clinical Preparation: Writing Activity

 15 minutes

1. What topics would you include in discharge instructions after hospitalization with bronchiolitis?

Copyright © 2007 by Saunders, an imprint of Elsevier Inc. All rights reserved.

2. These topics represent the content that must be taught. What about the methods you will use? What will you do to ensure that teaching is understood?

3. Providing anticipatory guidance is very important. Carrie Richards is 3½ months old. Identify some developmental changes her mother should anticipate in the next few weeks.

4. The only vaccine Carrie Richards has received is for hepatitis B. What teaching does Carrie Richards' mother need with regard to immunizations?

5. What if Carrie Richards' mother expresses concern about pain (she knows she avoids inflicting pain and perceives that the immunizations are painful)? How would you respond?

Copyright © 2007 by Saunders, an imprint of Elsevier Inc. All rights reserved.

6. In response to Carrie Richards' mother's concerns about pain, she may be given a prescription for EMLA cream to be used before her next well-child visit. What should the nurse tell her about its use?

Great job on completing this lesson! This content will help you to think about other related pediatric situations in the hospital setting.

Copyright © 2007 by Saunders, an imprint of Elsevier Inc. All rights reserved.

Caring for an Infant Who Is Failing to Thrive

 Reading Assignment: Health Promotion for the Developing Child
(Chapter 4, pages 91-94)
Health Promotion for the Infant (Chapter 5, pages 111-121)
The Child with a Psychosocial Disorder
(Chapter 29, pages 990-993)

Patient: Carrie Richards, Room 303

Objectives:

- Discuss the nutritional needs of the infant.
- Define *failure to thrive (FTT)*.
- Consider patterns of growth that may indicate FTT.
- Determine areas of assessment when FTT is suspected.
- Discuss the relationship of parenting skills to FTT.
- Develop specific interventions for caring for an infant with FTT.

As you complete this lesson, you will be exploring the complexities of care for failure to thrive, including the factors of parent-infant interaction and parenting skills. You will consider the role of the nurse in assessment, support, and teaching when providing care in the case of failure to thrive.

Exercise 1

Clinical Preparation: Writing Activity

15 minutes

1. Why is adequate nutrition so important in infancy?

77

Copyright © 2007 by Saunders, an imprint of Elsevier Inc. All rights reserved.

2. What should Carrie Richards' nutritional intake be like at 3½ months of age?

3. Differentiate between organic and nonorganic failure to thrive.

4. The following is a lengthy list of assessment data. Some data are physiologic, and some are psychosocial. Which of the following should be assessed when there is a concern about failure to thrive? Select all that apply.

_____ Weight less than 5th percentile

_____ Sudden deceleration in growth

_____ Delay in reaching milestones

_____ Decreased muscle mass

_____ Muscle hypotonia

_____ Abdominal distention

_____ General weakness

_____ Cachexia

_____ Avoidance of eye contact or touch

_____ Intense watchfulness

_____ Sleep disturbance

_____ Lack of age-appropriate stranger anxiety

_____ Lack of preference for parents

_____ Repetitive self-stimulating behavior

Copyright © 2007 by Saunders, an imprint of Elsevier Inc. All rights reserved.

5. What are the potential long-term effects of untreated failure to thrive?

Exercise 2

 CD-ROM Activity

 30 minutes

- Sign in to work at Pacific View Regional Hospital for Period of Care 2. (*Note:* If you are already in the virtual hospital from a previous exercise, click on **Leave the Floor** and then **Restart the Program** to get to the sign-in window.)
- From the Patient List, select Carrie Richards (Room 303).
- Click on **Go to Nurses' Station**.
- Click on **Chart** and then on **303**.
- Click on and review the **Nursing Admission** tab.

 1. Review Carrie Richards' chart for growth information. Plot her length and weight on the growth chart found on page 1041 in your textbook. In what percentile does she fall? Does this assessment help you to see where there is a problem? Can you now visualize what Carrie looks like?

2. If you knew Carrie Richards' birth weight, how would you use the data? What is the expected weight gain for an infant at 6 months? At 12 months?

 - Now click on **Consultations**.
- Review the Dietary/Nutrition Consult.

3. Find Carrie Richards' birth weight. Based on this information, what concerns do you have about her rate of growth?

Copyright © 2007 by Saunders, an imprint of Elsevier Inc. All rights reserved.

4. You have considered the recommended diet for a 3½-month-old in question 2 of Exercise 1 in this lesson. How does this compare with Carrie Richards' actual diet? Evaluate the adequacy of her diet and consider her mother's rationales for these choices. Is there anything else you would like to know or assess?

➔ • Sometimes food allergies are a factor in failure to thrive. Review Carrie Richards' records, especially the **History and Physical** and **Consultations**.

5. Is there any evidence of a food allergy being a factor in Carrie's failure to thrive?

6. Based on your review of the Dietary/Nutrition Consult, what do you think is the problem in regard to Carrie Richards' feedings? What additional dietary recommendations are planned for her?

7. As you talk with Carrie Richards' mother, you learn that income is a problem. When discussing feedings, what should you incorporate in your teaching?

Copyright © 2007 by Saunders, an imprint of Elsevier Inc. All rights reserved.

8. How would you implement teaching about formula preparation for Carrie Richards' mother?

9. What are some other teaching priorities for Carrie Richards' mother?

10. Discuss interdisciplinary collaboration as it relates to Carrie Richards' failure to thrive. Who needs to be involved?

Exercise 3

 CD-ROM Activity

 30 minutes

- Sign in to work at Pacific View Regional Hospital for Period of Care 1. (*Note:* If you are already in the virtual hospital from a previous exercise, click on **Leave the Floor** and then **Restart the Program** to get to the sign-in window.)
- From the Patient List, select Carrie Richards (Room 303).
- Click on **Go to Nurses' Station**.
- Click on **Chart** and then on **303**.
- Click on and review the **History and Physical** tab.

Copyright © 2007 by Saunders, an imprint of Elsevier Inc. All rights reserved.

1. In the previous exercise, you considered the following assessment data in regard to failure to thrive. Which of these specifically apply to Carrie Richards? Select all that apply.

_____ Weight less than 5th percentile

_____ Sudden deceleration in growth

_____ Delay in reaching milestones

_____ Decreased muscle mass

_____ Muscle hypotonia

_____ Abdominal distention

_____ General weakness

_____ Cachexia

_____ Avoidance of eye contact or touch

_____ Intense watchfulness

_____ Sleep disturbance

_____ Lack of age-appropriate stranger anxiety

_____ Lack of preference for parents

_____ Repetitive self-stimulating behaviors

2. What are some risk factors in Carrie Richards' situation?

- Click on **Return to Nurses' Station** and then on **303**.
- Click on **Patient Care** and then on **Nurse-Client Interactions**.
- Select and view the video titled **0755: Intervention—Weight**. (*Note:* Check the virtual clock to see whether enough time has elapsed. You can use the fast-forward feature to advance the time by 2-minute intervals if the video is not yet available. Then click again on **Patient Care** and **Nurse-Client Interactions** to refresh the screen.)

3. How should the nurse weigh Carrie Richards? Why has she elected to obtain the weight before feeding? After all, Carrie has been fussy and seems to want to be fed.

Copyright © 2007 by Saunders, an imprint of Elsevier Inc. All rights reserved.

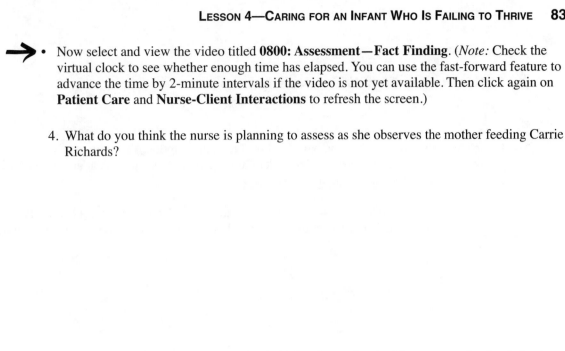

→ • Now select and view the video titled **0800: Assessment—Fact Finding**. (*Note:* Check the virtual clock to see whether enough time has elapsed. You can use the fast-forward feature to advance the time by 2-minute intervals if the video is not yet available. Then click again on **Patient Care** and **Nurse-Client Interactions** to refresh the screen.)

4. What do you think the nurse is planning to assess as she observes the mother feeding Carrie Richards?

5. Why is it essential to know that Carrie Richards' mother is able to respond to her infant's cues and correctly interpret them?

6. Are there other areas you would like to explore in this situation? If so, what are they?

7. Suppose that Carrie Richards' mother says, "Can't you just change the formula? I don't understand why we need all these tests." How should the nurse respond?

Copyright © 2007 by Saunders, an imprint of Elsevier Inc. All rights reserved.

Exercise 4

Clinical Preparation: Writing Activity

15 minutes

Review the Nursing Care Plan on pages 991-993 in your textbook. This care plan addresses growth in the infant as well as knowledge deficit in the parent. Pay particular attention to the areas of ongoing assessment and monitoring.

1. Based on what you have learned in previous exercises, what other nursing diagnosis might be appropriate for Carrie Richards' mother? (*Hint:* Consider the lack of resources available to her.)

2. Create a short-term goal with specific outcome criteria that is related to this nursing diagnosis.

3. Develop nursing interventions to help achieve the criteria you identified in question 2.

4. Write an evaluative statement that reflects meeting the goal you created in question 2.

Copyright © 2007 by Saunders, an imprint of Elsevier Inc. All rights reserved.

Exercise 5

 Clinical Preparation: Writing Activity

15 minutes

1. What if you noticed that Carrie Richards' mother always had the TV on while feeding her and seemed to pay more attention to the TV than to Carrie? How would you intervene?

 2. Refer to pages 982-988 in your textbook. The definition of *child abuse* refers to emotional abuse, physical abuse, and neglect. Is there evidence of abuse in this situation? Is there a risk for abuse? Share your thoughts.

Copyright © 2007 by Saunders, an imprint of Elsevier Inc. All rights reserved.

3. Envision yourself working with Carrie Richards' mother. How do you feel toward her? What do you think it would be like to carry out the teaching plans articulated (most particularly for the deficient knowledge nursing diagnosis on pages 988-989)? (*Hint:* Think about what the term *rescue fantasy* means to you.)

4. Identify and discuss your own biases about child abuse and neglect.

5. What is the nurse's responsibility in a suspected case of child abuse?

Great work! Having completed this lesson, you have confronted a challenging nursing care problem and have started to look at supporting strengths as well as recognizing problems where other collaboration needs to occur.

Copyright © 2007 by Saunders, an imprint of Elsevier Inc. All rights reserved.

LESSON **5**

The Young Child in the Hospital

/OD **Reading Assignment:** Health Promotion for the Developing Child
(Chapter 4, pages 63-72, 79-95)
Health Promotion During Early Childhood
(Chapter 6, pages 135-162)
The Ill Child in the Hospital and Other Care Settings
(Chapter 11, pages 288-291, 293-304)

Patient: Stephanie Brown, Room 304

Objectives:

- Identify developmental milestones for early childhood.
- Score a DDST II on a young child and discuss the implications for promoting development.
- Discuss common fears and care needs of the young child who is hospitalized.
- Determine nursing interventions necessary for promoting development in the young child who is hospitalized.
- Identify areas for anticipatory guidance to be provided for the parents of a young child.
- Discuss parental needs while a young child is hospitalized.

In this lesson you will be caring for a young child who is hospitalized and whose mother is present. You will learn how to consider growth and development when providing care for this child. This includes consideration of a child who is transitioning from one developmental stage to another and who may be displaying characteristics of each stage. You will also learn how to anticipate and be responsive to the needs of the parent.

Copyright © 2007 by Saunders, an imprint of Elsevier Inc. All rights reserved.

Exercise 1

 Clinical Preparation: Writing Activity

45 minutes

1. Describe the pattern of physical growth during the toddler and preschool periods.

2. Envision observing a 2-year-old and a 5-year-old. Given your knowledge of physical growth and development, describe the differences in their physical appearances.

3. Below, compare and contrast the toddler and preschool periods by giving an example for each aspect of development listed.

Aspect of Development	Toddler	Preschooler
Gross/fine motor development		
Cognitive/sensory development		
Language skills		
Psychosocial development		

Copyright © 2007 by Saunders, an imprint of Elsevier Inc. All rights reserved.

4. Describe the play behaviors expected for toddlers as compared with preschoolers.

5. What is Erikson's developmental task for the toddler? Describe its meaning in your own words, as if you were explaining the task to a parent.

6. What is Erikson's developmental task for the preschooler? Describe its meaning in your own words, as if you were explaining the task to a parent.

7. One area of development for the preschooler is that of fine motor skills. Which activity would best promote this type of skill development?
   a. Playing house
   b. Cutting and pasting
   c. Sand play
   d. Throwing a ball

8. Freud's theory of psychosexual development is relevant during the preschool period. What is the major task Freud addresses for the toddler? For the preschooler?

Copyright © 2007 by Saunders, an imprint of Elsevier Inc. All rights reserved.

9. Review Piaget's description of preoperational thought. Explain how this might be considered in the care of the hospitalized child.

10. Anticipate taking care of a young child in the hospital. What nursing interventions would facilitate a positive experience for the toddler?

11. What nursing interventions would facilitate a positive experience for the preschooler?

Copyright © 2007 by Saunders, an imprint of Elsevier Inc. All rights reserved.

12. Define regression and provide a common example of it for the toddler and an example for the preschooler.

Exercise 2

 CD-ROM Activity

 30 minutes

- Sign in to work at Pacific View Regional Hospital for Period of Care 1. (*Note:* If you are already in the virtual hospital from a previous exercise, click on **Leave the Floor** and then **Restart the Program** to get to the sign-in window.)
- From the Patient List, select Stephanie Brown (Room 304).
- Click on **Go to Nurses' Station**.
- Click on **Chart** and then on **304**.
- Click on and review the **History and Physical** tab.
- Click on and review other areas of the chart as needed for additional information.

1. Select evidence of growth and development from Stephanie Brown's chart and record it in the appropriate location in the table below.

Area of Development	Stephanie Brown's Growth and Development
Gross/fine motor skill development	
Cognitive/sensory development	
Language skills	
Psychosocial development	

Copyright © 2007 by Saunders, an imprint of Elsevier Inc. All rights reserved.

2. Using the DDST II found on the textbook's Evolve website, plot the information you have and summarize Stephanie Brown's development as you see it. (*Hint:* You will need to determine her exact age in months.)

 3. Stephanie Brown has cerebral palsy. What aspects of her development might be most affected as a young child with cerebral palsy? What aspects of her development might be affected in the future? (*Hint:* See pages 939-940 in your textbook for a discussion of cerebral palsy.)

Copyright © 2007 by Saunders, an imprint of Elsevier Inc. All rights reserved.

4. Develop strategies to support the needs of a hospitalized child between the age of 2 and 5 years.

5. Discuss teaching opportunities to promote growth and development for the child described in question 4.

 • Click on **Return to Nurses' Station** and then on **304**.

• Click on **Patient Care** and then on **Nurse-Client Interactions**.

• Select and view the video **0730: Assessment—Neuro Status**. (*Note:* Check the virtual clock to see whether enough time has elapsed. You can use the fast-forward feature to advance the time by 2-minute intervals if the video is not yet available. Then click again on **Patient Care** and **Nurse-Client Interactions** to refresh the screen.)

Copyright © 2007 by Saunders, an imprint of Elsevier Inc. All rights reserved.

6. What needs does Stephanie Brown's mother have? How can the nurse support her?

- Click on **Chart** and then on **304**.
- Click on the **History and Physical** tab.
- Review Stephanie's immunization status.

7. Are Stephanie Brown's immunizations up to date? Identify the immunizations she should have had by age 3 years.

Exercise 3

Clinical Preparation: Writing Activity

15 minutes

1. Respond to this statement: "Hospitalization can still be a time of growth."

Copyright © 2007 by Saunders, an imprint of Elsevier Inc. All rights reserved.

2. What is meant by the statement "Play is a child's work"?

3. Create a scenario in which you might anticipate using some of the above thinking in your care of young children.

You are now ready to consider and use all of this information as you take care of Stephanie and provide nursing care for her acute illness.

Copyright © 2007 by Saunders, an imprint of Elsevier Inc. All rights reserved.

Caring for a Young Child with Meningitis

∽⧔ **Reading Assignment:** Principles and Procedures for Nursing Care of Children
(Chapter 13, pages 352, 354)
The Child with a Neurologic Alteration
(Chapter 28, pages 922, 953-956)

Patient: Stephanie Brown, Room 304

Objectives:

- Describe the pathophysiology of meningitis.
- Discuss risk factors for meningitis.
- List assessment data indicative of meningitis.
- Explain the rationale for the treatment of meningitis.
- Develop a care plan for a child with meningitis.
- Discuss strategies for supporting a parent and child through diagnosis and treatment.

In this lesson you will learn about the problem of meningitis in a child, along with related nursing care. You will focus on a variety of challenges associated with this disorder. You may need to review the concepts of growth and development of a young child, as well as teaching-learning principles.

Copyright © 2007 by Saunders, an imprint of Elsevier Inc. All rights reserved.

Exercise 1

 CD-ROM Activity

 45 minutes

1. Review the information on the pathophysiology of meningitis on page 954 of your text-book. Explain the pathophysiology in terms that a parent could understand.

 • Sign in to work at Pacific View Regional Hospital for Period of Care 1. (*Note:* If you are already in the virtual hospital from a previous exercise, click on **Leave the Floor** and then **Restart the Program** to get to the sign-in window.)
   • From the Patient List, select Stephanie Brown (Room 304).
   • Click on **Get Report** and read the clinical report.
   • Click on **Go to Nurses' Station**.
   • Click on **Chart** and then on **304**.
   • Click on and review the following sections: **Physician's Notes**, **History and Physical**, **Nursing Admission**, and **Emergency Department**.

Copyright © 2007 by Saunders, an imprint of Elsevier Inc. All rights reserved.

2. Given the information you have learned about Stephanie Brown and her family, reflect on your response to question 1. Would you change anything? If your answer is yes, what would you change and how would you present the information? If the answer is no, identify the strengths reflected in your teaching about the medical diagnosis. Make sure your response reflects some of the information you have learned that affects teaching in this situation. Incorporate other teaching-learning principles as they apply.

3. What in Stephanie Brown's situation increases her risk for developing meningitis?

4. What assessment data did Stephanie Brown exhibit on admission that would indicate a diagnosis of meningitis?

5. What additional assessments would you like to make?

Copyright © 2007 by Saunders, an imprint of Elsevier Inc. All rights reserved.

6. If Stephanie Brown were an infant and had this diagnosis, what additional assessments would you perform?

7. In addition to nuchal rigidity, positive responses to two other signs were elicited from

Stephanie Brown that are indicative of meningitis. They are _____

and _____ signs.

8. Explain how each of the signs listed below are tested. Then briefly describe the response that each sign would elicit in a child with meningitis.

Sign	Test	Response in Meningitis
Nuchal rigidity		
Kernig's sign		
Brudzinski's sign		

→ • Click on and review the **Physician's Orders** and **Diagnostic Reports**.

9. What test is diagnostic for meningitis? What data are consistent with a diagnosis of meningitis?

Copyright © 2007 by Saunders, an imprint of Elsevier Inc. All rights reserved.

10. How would you anticipate supporting Stephanie Brown through the procedure of lumbar puncture?

11. Given that increased intracranial pressure is a possibility in a child with meningitis, what changes in vital signs would be significant?

12. Discuss the types of meningitis most commonly seen in childhood. Incorporate etiologic factors in your answer.

13. Which type of meningitis is associated with droplet transmission and increased risk for infection as exposure to contacts expands?

14. Match each of the following physician's orders with its rationale.

Physician's Order	Rationale
_____ Pulse oximetry q4h	a. Provides a baseline (aminoglycosides can cause ototoxicity)
_____ Neuro checks q4h	b. To reduce intracranial pressure (by gravity)
_____ Blood culture for fever above 101 degrees	c. To monitor therapeutic blood level
_____ Audiogram	d. Monitoring of neurologic status
_____ Keep HOB elevated 45 degrees	e. To avoid transmission via droplets
_____ Respiratory isolation	f. Assessment for other causative agents
_____ Vancomycin levels	g. Ongoing monitoring of O_2 status

Copyright © 2007 by Saunders, an imprint of Elsevier Inc. All rights reserved.

Exercise 2

 CD-ROM Activity

 60 minutes

- Sign in to work at Pacific View Regional Hospital Period of Care 1. (*Note:* If you are already in the virtual hospital from a previous exercise, click on **Leave the Floor** and then **Restart the Program** to get to the sign-in window.)
- From the Patient List, select Stephanie Brown (Room 304).
- Click on **Go to Nurses' Station** and then on **304**.
- Click on **Patient Care** and complete a focused assessment of Stephanie Brown's neurologic status.
- When you finish your assessment, click on **Leave the Floor**.
- From the Floor Menu, select **Look at Your Preceptor's Evaluations**.
- Next, click on **Examination Report** and review the feedback.

1. Reflect on your assessment skills. Did you miss any areas?

- Click on **Return to Evaluations** and then **Return to Menu**.
- From the Floor Menu, click on **Restart the Program**.
- Sign in to work at Pacific View Regional Hospital for Period of Care 1.
- From the Patient List, select Stephanie Brown (Room 304).
- Click on **Go to Nurses' Station**.
- Click on **Chart** and then on **304**.
- Click on the **Emergency Department** tab and check Stephanie's admission vital signs.
- Next, click on **Return to Nurses' Station** and then on **304**.
- Click on **Take Vitals Signs**.

Copyright © 2007 by Saunders, an imprint of Elsevier Inc. All rights reserved.

2. How do Stephanie's current vital signs compare with those taken in the ED? Do you have concerns about increased intracranial pressure?

- Click on **Leave the Floor**.
- Click on **Restart the Program**.
- Sign in to work at Pacific View Regional Hospital for Period of Care 2.
- From the Patient List, select Stephanie Brown.
- Click on **Go to Nurses' Station** and then on **304**.
- Click on **Patient Care** and then on **Nurse-Client Interactions**.
- Select and view the video titled **1120: Preventing Spread of Disease**. (*Note:* Check the virtual clock to see whether enough time has elapsed. You can use the fast-forward feature to advance the time by 2-minute intervals if the video is not yet available. Then click again on **Patient Care** and **Nurse-Client Interactions** to refresh the screen.)

3. What kind of isolation was the nurse in the video observing? Was this correct and consistent with the physician's orders?

4. CDC guidelines require standard precautions for all types of meningitis, as well as droplet precautions for certain types. What else needs to be included to implement droplet precautions effectively? (*Hint:* Read the information about standard precautions found on your textbook's Evolve website.)

Copyright © 2007 by Saunders, an imprint of Elsevier Inc. All rights reserved.

5. The above guidelines are implemented immediately and kept in place until 24 hours after antibiotics have been started. Antibiotics are always administered before cultures come back. Why is that?

6. Suppose that you see Stephanie Brown's mother not wearing a mask. When you ask her about this, she says she doesn't need to do anything special because she never leaves Stephanie Brown's room. How would you respond?

→ • Now select and view the video titled **1145: Teaching—Disease Sequelae**. (*Note:* Check the virtual clock to see whether enough time has elapsed. You can use the fast-forward feature to advance the time by 2-minute intervals if the video is not yet available. Then click again on **Patient Care** and **Nurse-Client Interactions** to refresh the screen.)

7. Discuss the most common potential sequelae associated with meningitis. Incorporate the mechanism of injury in your answer.

8. Is Stephanie Brown on any treatment or medication that may contribute to permanent injury?

Copyright © 2007 by Saunders, an imprint of Elsevier Inc. All rights reserved.

• Click on **Chart** and then on **304**.
  • Click on and review the **Physician's Orders** tab.

9. Review Stephanie Brown's IV orders. Calculate the total volume for 24 hours.

 • Click on **Return to Room 304**.
  • Click on **Leave the Floor** and then **Restart the Program**.
  • Sign in to work at Pacific View Regional Hospital for Period of Care 3.
  • From the Patient List, select Stephanie Brown.
  • Click on **Go to Nurses' Station** and then on **304**.
  • Click on **Patient Care** and then **Nurse-Client Interactions**.
  • Select and view the video titled **1510: Nurse-Patient Communication**. (*Note:* Check the virtual clock to see whether enough time has elapsed. You can use the fast-forward feature to advance the time by 2-minute intervals if the video is not yet available. Then click again on **Patient Care** and **Nurse-Client Interactions** to refresh the screen.)

10. What is the nurse's assessment and decision during this interaction?

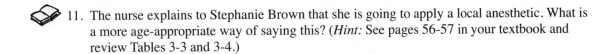 11. The nurse explains to Stephanie Brown that she is going to apply a local anesthetic. What is a more age-appropriate way of saying this? (*Hint:* See pages 56-57 in your textbook and review Tables 3-3 and 3-4.)

12. What is the anesthetic being used? How is it used in order to be most effective? (*Hint:* You may want to refer to a nursing drug handbook for complete information.)

Copyright © 2007 by Saunders, an imprint of Elsevier Inc. All rights reserved.

13. Note the nurse's interaction with Stephanie Brown and her mother. Why is Stephanie Brown, who is only 3 years old, included in the explanation?

14. At Stephanie Brown's age, how might she perceive her hospital experience? How might she perceive the nurse?

15. Consider the behavior of Stephanie Brown's mother. How might that affect Stephanie's perceptions?

16. From a developmental perspective, what are major fears of children in Stephanie Brown's age group? What behaviors might the child display?

Copyright © 2007 by Saunders, an imprint of Elsevier Inc. All rights reserved.

17. What strategies can you use to promote a more positive experience for Stephanie Brown while she is in the hospital?

There are medications ordered for Stephanie Brown, and you will be giving those medications to her in Lesson 18. If you would like to administer her medications, you can proceed to Lesson 18, Exercise 2.

Exercise 3

 Clinical Preparation: Writing Activity

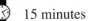 15 minutes

1. Explain the issue of prophylaxis for anyone who has had close contact with a patient who has meningitis.

2. Think about how you might respond to any questions that Stephanie Brown's daycare provider might have. What issues should be discussed?

3. What drug is used for prophylaxis of Haemophilus influenzae, and what particular information should be shared with the recipient?

Copyright © 2007 by Saunders, an imprint of Elsevier Inc. All rights reserved.

4. Let's assume that Stephanie Brown has had a relapse and is now doing worse. Other family members have been taking turns staying with her. She still has an IV and is very restless and irritable. Even the family members are getting irritable, and they have noticed all the babies on the unit that have to be fed and cared for. They worry about Stephanie Brown receiving the care she needs. How will you help them?

5. Every time you walk into the room wearing your mask, Stephanie starts to scream. On the other hand, when you see her through the window while you are not wearing the mask, she is willing to wave to you as she plays quietly with her mother. What is going on and how might you respond?

Now, move on to the next lesson and consider care of a chronic health problem and its impact on the child and family.

Copyright © 2007 by Saunders, an imprint of Elsevier Inc. All rights reserved.

Caring for a Young Child with Cerebral Palsy

Reading Assignment: Health Promotion for the Developing Child
(Chapter 4, pages 80-83)
The Child with a Neurologic Alteration
(Chapter 28, pages 939-942)

Patient: Stephanie Brown, Room 304

Objectives:

- Describe the behaviors and problems associated with the most common types of cerebral palsy (CP).
- Discuss a range of etiologic factors associated with cerebral palsy.
- Explain the importance of early diagnosis and treatment for the child's optimal level of functioning.
- Discuss the nursing care needs of a child with cerebral palsy and the family.

Completing this lesson will help you gain an appreciation of the challenges associated with caring for a child who has cerebral palsy—both for parents and for the nurse. You will also explore the issue of cerebral palsy as a coexisting condition when a different health problem is the primary reason for hospitalization or other health care encounter.

Copyright © 2007 by Saunders, an imprint of Elsevier Inc. All rights reserved.

Exercise 1

 CD-ROM Activity

 30 minutes

- Sign in to work at Pacific View Regional Hospital for Period of Care 1. (*Note:* If you are already in the virtual hospital from a previous exercise, click on **Leave the Floor** and then **Restart the Program** to get to the sign-in window.)
- From the Patient List, select Stephanie Brown (Room 304).
- Click on **Get Report** and read the clinical report.

1. Perhaps you have encountered children with cerebral palsy in your personal and/or professional experiences and remember thinking that these children seem challenging to care for. What is cerebral palsy?

2. What types of fine and gross motor functions may be affected by cerebral palsy?

 • Click on **Go to Nurses' Station** and then on **304**.
- Click on **Patient Care** and perform a focused assessment.

Copyright © 2007 by Saunders, an imprint of Elsevier Inc. All rights reserved.

3. Based on your assessment of Stephanie Brown, list any behavioral responses she demonstrates that are associated with CP.

- Click on **Chart** and then on **304**.
- Click on and review the **History and Physical** tab.

4. Review Stephanie Brown's history. What might be some etiologic factors for Stephanie Brown's cerebral palsy?

5. Early recognition and treatment are important to fostering achievement of optimal development. Why is cerebral palsy often not diagnosed until about 2 years of age?

- Click on **Return to Room 304**.
- Click on **Patient Care** and then on **Nurse-Client Interactions**.
- Select and view the video titled **0750: Caring for the Child with CP**. (*Note:* Check the virtual clock to see whether enough time has elapsed. You can use the fast-forward feature to advance the time by 2-minute intervals if the video is not yet available. Then click again on **Patient Care** and **Nurse-Client Interactions** to refresh the screen.)

6. What is the nurse assessing as she listens to Stephanie Brown's mother explain Stephanie's problems associated with cerebral palsy?

Copyright © 2007 by Saunders, an imprint of Elsevier Inc. All rights reserved.

7. Should the nurse be supportive of the mother's home treatments and strategies? Why or why not?

8. For what problem is Stephanie Brown at risk during her hospitalization? (*Hint:* You will need to consider her developmental age.)

 • Click on **Chart** and then on **304**.
 • Click on the **Nursing Admission** tab and review the data concerning Stephanie Brown's development.

9. Hospitalization can be a time of growth. Explore the developmental tasks that Stephanie Brown has achieved and those she has not. Comment on her development.

 10. This is a good opportunity to explore Stephanie Brown's development further. Assume that she has recently turned 3 years of age. Using the DDST II score sheet found on the textbook's Evolve website, determine one skill that Stephanie should have completed, one that she is working on, and one that she is not yet ready for. Do this in one of the four skill areas. (*Hint:* You may first want to review how to use the DDST II on pages 80-83 of your textbook.)

Copyright © 2007 by Saunders, an imprint of Elsevier Inc. All rights reserved.

Exercise 2

 CD-ROM Activity

 30 minutes

- Sign in to work at Pacific View Regional Hospital for Period of Care 3. (*Note:* If you are already in the virtual hospital from a previous exercise, click on **Leave the Floor** and then **Restart the Program** to get to the sign-in window.)
- From the Patient List, select Stephanie Brown (Room 304).
- Click on **Get Report** and read the clinical report.
- Click on **Go to Nurses' Station**.
- Click on **Chart** and then on **304**.
- Click on and review the **History and Physical** tab.

1. Match each type of cerebral palsy with its description.

Type	Description
_____ Spastic	a. Rigid flexor and extensor muscles; tremors
_____ Dyskinetic/athetoid	b. Increased deep tendon reflexes, hypertonia, flexion, and scissors gait
_____ Ataxic	c. Slow, writhing uncontrolled and involuntary movements
_____ Rigid	d. Loss of coordination, equilibrium, and kinesthetic sense

2. What type of cerebral palsy does Stephanie Brown have? What are the signs that she manifests?

3. Cerebral palsy can have an impact on many aspects of the child's life. List several problems that can be associated with the behaviors the child manifests. (*Note:* Make sure that at least one is a psychosocial concern.)

Copyright © 2007 by Saunders, an imprint of Elsevier Inc. All rights reserved.

4. How would you respond if Stephanie Brown's mother expressed guilt over Stephanie's condition, saying that she knows now that she did some things that may have contributed to the condition? (*Hint:* You may want to review your response to question 4 in Exercise 1 of this lesson.)

5. In general, what is the etiology of cerebral palsy? What do these factors have in common?

6. Assume that Stephanie Brown's mother asks you whether you see any signs of mental retardation in her daughter. She is worried that this will develop as Stephanie's disease progresses. What can you tell her? How will you reassure her?

 • Click on **Return to Nurses' Station** and then on **304**.

• Click on **Patient Care** and then on **Nurse-Client Interactions**.

• Select and view the video titled **1530: Preventive Measures**. (*Note:* Check the virtual clock to see whether enough time has elapsed. You can use the fast-forward feature to advance the time by 2-minute intervals if the video is not yet available. Then click again on **Patient Care** and **Nurse-Client Interactions** to refresh the screen.)

7. Why does Stephanie Brown require heel cord stretching?

Copyright © 2007 by Saunders, an imprint of Elsevier Inc. All rights reserved.

8. What other preventive measures have been integrated into Stephanie Brown's regimen to prevent complications associated with cerebral palsy?

9. What is the nursing role with regard to supporting these preventive measures?

10. Explain why nutrition is so important for the child who has cerebral palsy.

11. Nurses are frequently asked for advice. Stephanie Brown's mother sends her daughter to a preschool program but wonders whether it is the best school for her. What advice can you give her?

Copyright © 2007 by Saunders, an imprint of Elsevier Inc. All rights reserved.

Exercise 3

Clinical Preparation: Writing Activity

30 minutes

1. When children are hospitalized for an acute illness, you may find that the child also has some other disability or chronic illness that could have an effect on the hospitalization or your care. Think about how you would provide care in such a situation. How do you get information? Who is in charge? Do you involve parents in the same ways you usually do? How do you feel about people with disabilities? Reflect and respond.

2. Develop a plan to teach Stephanie Brown's mother to promote self-esteem as Stephanie progresses through the stage of initiative versus guilt. First, write one or more goals.

3. Now develop nursing interventions designed to meet the goal(s) you identified in question 2. (*Hint:* See Table 3-5 on page 59 in your textbook. Some of these examples can be adapted.)

Copyright © 2007 by Saunders, an imprint of Elsevier Inc. All rights reserved.

4. Does your community have a Children with Special Health Care Needs Program or an Early Intervention Program? What do you think these programs are about?

5. Visit www.ucp.org and then respond to the following questions:

a. What did you like or not like about this website?

b. To whom is this site geared?

c. What new information did you learn from this website?

Copyright © 2007 by Saunders, an imprint of Elsevier Inc. All rights reserved.

d. Would you recommend this website to parents of a child with cerebral palsy? Why or why not?

Great job! In addition to nursing care for a child with a chronic health problem, you have also learned to recognize the collaborative role you might have with parents in the care of their children.

Copyright © 2007 by Saunders, an imprint of Elsevier Inc. All rights reserved.

LESSON 8

The Hospitalized School-Age Child

📖 **Reading Assignment:** Health Promotion for the Developing Child
(Chapter 4, pages 63-79, 86-95)
Health Promotion for the School-Age Child
(Chapter 7, pages 164-184)
The Ill Child in the Hospital and Other Care Settings
(Chapter 11, pages 288, 291-292)

Patient: George Gonzalez, Room 301

Objectives:

- Discuss major growth and development events occurring during the school-age period.
- Contrast physical and psychosocial growth and development for a 6-year-old and a 12-year-old.
- Identify and discuss developmental tasks as defined by Erikson, Piaget, and Kohlberg.
- Discuss developmentally appropriate approaches for caring for the hospitalized school-aged child.

In this lesson you will be exploring the wide range of growth and development in the school-age years. Through your activities you will appreciate the child's abilities to take on more aspects of self-care and personal responsibility.

Copyright © 2007 by Saunders, an imprint of Elsevier Inc. All rights reserved.

Exercise 1

Clinical Preparation: Writing Activity

30 minutes

1. What are the major physical developmental changes for the school-age period?

2. What is Erikson's task for the school-age period?

3. Provide some examples of school activities that promote growth and development.

4. Using Piaget's theory, describe the sequence of cognitive development during the school-age period.

Copyright © 2007 by Saunders, an imprint of Elsevier Inc. All rights reserved.

5. Explain how cognitive development affects coping with hospitalization.

6. Describe Kohlberg's stages of moral development as they relate to the school-age child.

7. Describe the evolution of social development and peer relationships throughout the school-age period.

8. Identify strategies to help a school-age child cope with hospitalization. Choose a young, middle, or older school-age child.

Copyright © 2007 by Saunders, an imprint of Elsevier Inc. All rights reserved.

Exercise 2

 CD-ROM Activity

 45 minutes

- Sign in to work at Pacific View Regional Hospital for Period of Care 1. (*Note:* If you are already in the virtual hospital from a previous exercise, click on **Leave the Floor** and then **Restart the Program** to get to the sign-in window.
- From the Patient List, select George Gonzalez (Room 301).
- Click on **Go to Nurses' Station**.
- Click on **Chart** and then on **301**.
- Click on and review the **History and Physical** tab.

1. What information on growth and development did you find in your review of George Gonzalez's chart?

2. Discuss any areas that are abnormal or present a "red flag" for you.

 • Click on **Return to Nurses' Station** and then on **301**.
- Click on **Patient Care** and then on **Nurse-Client Interactions**.
- Select and view the video titled **0730: Supervision—Glucose Testing**. (*Note:* Check the virtual clock to see whether enough time has elapsed. You can use the fast-forward feature to advance the time by 2-minute intervals if the video is not yet available. Then click again on **Patient Care** and **Nurse-Client Interactions** to refresh the screen.)

Copyright © 2007 by Saunders, an imprint of Elsevier Inc. All rights reserved.

3. What physical development skills is George Gonzalez using?

4. What cognitive skills does he need?

5. What does the nurse do to foster self-esteem in George?

➜ • Once again, click on **Patient Care** and then on **Nurse-Client Interactions**.
   • Select and view the video titled **0745: Self-Administering Insulin**. (*Note:* Check the virtual clock to see whether enough time has elapsed. You can use the fast-forward feature to advance the time by 2-minute intervals if the video is not yet available. Then click again on **Patient Care** and **Nurse-Client Interactions** to refresh the screen.)

6. Identify the physical skills necessary for self-administration of insulin.

7. Identify the cognitive skills that George needs in order to be independent with this self-care skill.

8. Devise strategies to foster self-esteem as George Gonzalez learns self-care skills for diabetes management.

Copyright © 2007 by Saunders, an imprint of Elsevier Inc. All rights reserved.

9. What evidence suggests that George Gonzalez does or does not get enough exercise?

10. What areas of anticipatory guidance should the nurse discuss with George's mother?

Exercise 3

Clinical Preparation: Writing Activity

15 minutes

1. Define what is meant by latch-key or self-care children.

2. What suggestions can the nurse offer to the parent to increase safety and decrease parental guilt in the situation of care for latch-key children?

Copyright © 2007 by Saunders, an imprint of Elsevier Inc. All rights reserved.

3. Many schools are providing before- and after-school programs. What are some of the advantages of such programs?

4. Nurses may find that school-age children are already dealing with problems such as exposure to tobacco, drugs, and alcohol. Share your thoughts on how you might feel and respond in such a situation.

Copyright © 2007 by Saunders, an imprint of Elsevier Inc. All rights reserved.

Caring for a School-Age Child with Diabetes Mellitus

∽ **Reading Assignment:** The Child with an Endocrine or Metabolic Alteration
(Chapter 27, pages 898-915)

Patient: George Gonzalez, Room 301

Objectives:

- Discuss the pathophysiology of diabetes mellitus.
- Compare and contrast type 1 and type 2 diabetes mellitus.
- Explain the role of insulin in the metabolism of foods.
- Discuss management and nursing responsibilities for insulin therapy, diet, exercise, and blood glucose monitoring.
- Contrast causes, signs, and management of hypoglycemia and hyperglycemia.
- Explain the pathophysiology of diabetic ketoacidosis (DKA) and discuss its management and nursing care.
- Discuss the impact of growth and development on diabetes management.

Most likely, you have had instruction in diabetes and have a basic understanding of the disease and its problems. In this lesson you will work with 11-year-old George Gonzalez in Room 301. You will learn more about diabetes by considering problems and nursing care based on the current status of George's illness. In doing so, you will need to apply principles of growth and development. Although teaching may be touched on in this lesson, the teaching-learning process, as it relates to the care of the child with diabetes and his family, will be discussed in more depth in the next lesson.

Copyright © 2007 by Saunders, an imprint of Elsevier Inc. All rights reserved.

Exercise 1

Clinical Preparation: Writing Activity

30 minutes

1. Define *diabetes mellitus*.

2. What are some risk factors for developing diabetes mellitus?

3. Match each of the following characteristics to either type 1 or type 2 diabetes mellitus to show your understanding of the differences between these two conditions.

Characteristic	Type
_____ This is the most common childhood endocrine disease.	a. Type 1
_____ This type results from an autoimmune process disorder.	b. Type 2
_____ Cells are unable to use insulin.	
_____ Genetic predisposition is a factor.	
_____ Pancreas is unable to produce insulin.	
_____ Obesity commonly coexists.	

Copyright © 2007 by Saunders, an imprint of Elsevier Inc. All rights reserved.

4. What symptoms would a person newly diagnosed with diabetes manifest? (*Hint:* Be sure to consider growth and development in your discussion.)

5. What are the signs of hyperglycemia?

6. How is hyperglycemia treated?

7. What is the relationship between exercise and insulin?

Copyright © 2007 by Saunders, an imprint of Elsevier Inc. All rights reserved.

8. What are the signs of hypoglycemia?

9. How is hypoglycemia managed?

10. What is Hb_{A1C}? Explain its use as a diagnostic and teaching tool.

11. Most commonly, physicians order a combination of short-acting and intermediate-acting insulin to treat and manage diabetes mellitus. Match each type of insulin below with its corresponding characteristics.

Characteristic of Insulin	Type of Insulin
_____ Onset of 15-30 minutes	a. Regular
_____ Onset of 1-1½ hours	b. NPH
_____ Peaks at 5-10 hours	
_____ Peaks at 2-4 hours	
_____ Duration of 6-8 hours	
_____ Duration of 24 hours	

Copyright © 2007 by Saunders, an imprint of Elsevier Inc. All rights reserved.

Exercise 2

 CD-ROM Activity

 45 minutes

- Sign in to work at Pacific View Regional Hospital for Period of Care 1. (*Note:* If you are already in the virtual hospital from a previous exercise, click on **Leave the Floor** and then **Restart the Program** to get to the sign-in window.)
- From the Patient List, select George Gonzalez (Room 301).
- Click on **Go to Nurses' Station**.
- Click on **Chart** and then on **301**.
- Click on and review the **Emergency Department** tab.

1. What are the signs of diabetic ketoacidosis (DKA)?

2. Explain diabetic ketoacidosis.

3. What was George's condition when he was admitted? Was there a precipitating factor?

Copyright © 2007 by Saunders, an imprint of Elsevier Inc. All rights reserved.

4. What will be the focus of care for the first portion of George's hospitalization for DKA?

5. What type of insulin is used and why? Identify any nursing concerns associated with the administration of insulin IV.

 • Click on **Return to Nurses' Station** and then on **301**.
   • Click on **Patient Care** and then on **Physical Assessment**.
   • Complete a head-to-toe assessment.
   • Click on **Chart** and then on **301**.
   • Click on and review the **Emergency Department** and **Laboratory Reports** tabs.

6. Considering George's clinical situation, for which of the following nursing diagnoses is there evidence? Provide the data that led you to this choice.
   a. Fluid volume deficit related to abnormal fluid losses through diuresis and emesis.
   b. Risk for injury from altered acid-base balance leading to ketone production and acidosis related to lack of insulin.
   c. Knowledge deficit related to unfamiliarity with home management during sick days.

Copyright © 2007 by Saunders, an imprint of Elsevier Inc. All rights reserved.

7. What ongoing assessments need to be made when working with George Gonzalez?

8. What evidence is there that George's diabetes is out of control? How did he respond to treatment measures?

Let's take a step back and think about how George Gonzalez got here.

→ • Click on and review the **History and Physical** tab.

9. What factor in his history puts George at particular risk for developing diabetes?

10. When was George first diagnosed with diabetes?

11. What symptoms might George's mother have observed at the onset of his illness?

Copyright © 2007 by Saunders, an imprint of Elsevier Inc. All rights reserved.

• Click on **Return to Nurses' Station** and then on **301**.

- Click on **Patient Care** and then on **Nurse-Client Interactions**.

- Select and view the video titled **0730: Supervision—Glucose Testing**. (*Note:* Check the virtual clock to see whether enough time has elapsed. You can use the fast-forward feature to advance the time by 2-minute intervals if the video is not yet available. Then click again on **Patient Care** and **Nurse-Client Interactions** to refresh the screen.)

12. What did the nurse do that facilitated George's honesty about his testing skills and how he feels about them?

13. What is the nurse trying to accomplish when she asks George to do his own finger stick? (*Hint:* Consider developmental tasks of the school-age child.)

14. How might George's developmental stage affect his compliance with treatment plans?

 • Click on **Patient Care** and then on **Nurse-Client Interactions**.

- Select and view the video titled **0745: Self-Administering Insulin**. (*Note:* Check the virtual clock to see whether enough time has elapsed. You can use the fast-forward feature to advance the time by 2-minute intervals if the video is not yet available. Then click again on **Patient Care** and **Nurse-Client Interactions** to refresh the screen.)

15. What does the nurse do in this interaction that is positive as she observes George Gonzalez give his injection?

Copyright © 2007 by Saunders, an imprint of Elsevier Inc. All rights reserved.

Exercise 3

 CD-ROM Activity

 45 minutes

- Sign in to work at Pacific View Regional Hospital for Period of Care 1. (*Note:* If you are already in the virtual hospital from a previous exercise, click on **Leave the Floor** and then **Restart the Program** to get to the sign-in window.)
- From the Patient List, select George Gonzalez (Room 301).
- Click on **Go to Nurses' Station**.
- George needs insulin. Click on **MAR** to check the order for insulin.
- Click on **Return to Nurses' Station** and then on **301**.
- Before going to the Medication Room, complete any necessary assessments.
- Click on **Medication Room**.
- Using the Six Rights, prepare the correct dose of insulin for George Gonzalez. When you have prepared the medication, return to George's room and administer it, again following the Six Rights. (*Hint:* Try to perform these steps on your own. If you need help, refer to pages 26-30 and 37-41 in the **Getting Started** section of this workbook.)
- After administering the insulin, click on **Leave the Floor** and then **Look at Your Preceptor's Evaluations**.
- Next, click on **Medication Scorecard** and review the feedback.

  1. Identify the things you need to do, if any, to satisfactorily complete the procedure.

- Click on **Return to Evaluations** and then **Return to Menu**.
- Click on **Restart the Program**.
- Sign in to work at Pacific View Regional Hospital for for Period of Care 1.
- From the Patient List, select George Gonzalez (Room 301).
- Click on **Go to Nurses' Station**.
- Click on **Chart** and then on **301**.
- Click on the **Physician's Orders** tab. Find the order for George's morning dose of insulin.

  2. Using George's morning insulin order, describe the steps for drawing up two forms of insulin into one syringe.

Copyright © 2007 by Saunders, an imprint of Elsevier Inc. All rights reserved.

3. Explain why the procedure is done this way.

4. How should George Gonzalez be advised to rotate injection sites?

5. What are some possible barriers to compliance for George Gonzalez?

Let's review and reinforce your insulin administration skills.

- Click on **Leave the Floor** and then **Restart the Program**.
- Sign in to work at Pacific View Regional Hospital for Period of Care 1.
- From the Patient List, select George Gonzalez (Room 301).
- Click on **Go to Nurses' Station**.
- Once again, prepare and administer George's morning dose of insulin. Using the Six Rights, be sure to check the order, as well as George's blood glucose level. Perform the proper identification checks before giving the medication.
- After administering the insulin, check your performance by clicking on **Leave the Floor** and then on **Look at Your Preceptor's Evaluations**.
- Click on and review the **Medication Scorecard**.

6. Reflect on your performance. Consider the actual practice you may need in order to feel comfortable with this skill.

Copyright © 2007 by Saunders, an imprint of Elsevier Inc. All rights reserved.

7. List the possible learning needs of a patient newly diagnosed with diabetes.

8. Now refer to the list of learning needs on page 909 in your textbook. How did you do with your list in question 7? Consider any needs you left off your list. Are there any commonalities? Why do you think they were more difficult for you to remember?

9. Which of the above learning needs currently apply to George Gonzalez and his family?

Copyright © 2007 by Saunders, an imprint of Elsevier Inc. All rights reserved.

10. What anticipatory guidance can you offer George Gonzalez's mother with regard to how insulin needs change as George moves toward adolescence?

11. Discuss the relationships among insulin, food, and exercise. Explain them in terms that would be understandable by George Gonzalez and his family.

Let's jump ahead to visit George Gonzalez a little later in the day.

- Click on **Return to Evaluations**, **Return to Menu**, and **Restart the Program**.
- Sign in to work at Pacific View Regional Hospital for Period of Care 2.
- From the Patient List, select George Gonzalez (Room 301).
- Click on **Go to Nurses' Station** and then on **301**.
- Click on **Patient Care** and then on **Nurse-Client Interactions**.
- Select and view the video titled **1115: Teaching—Disease Process**. (*Note:* Check the virtual clock to see whether enough time has elapsed. You can use the fast-forward feature to advance the time by 2-minute intervals if the video is not yet available. Then click again on **Patient Care** and **Nurse-Client Interactions** to refresh the screen.)

12. What are the sequelae of untreated or poorly managed diabetes? Explain why they occur.

Copyright © 2007 by Saunders, an imprint of Elsevier Inc. All rights reserved.

Exercise 4

Clinical Preparation: Writing Activity

30 minutes

1. Treatment for diabetes is occurring more frequently on an outpatient basis. Why do you think this is happening? How can the outpatient or office nurse respond to learning needs of children such as George Gonzalez?

2. Compare and contrast two or more of the following websites designed for individuals with diabetes and their families. For each website that you choose, write about the target group, ease of use, and appropriateness for patients with diabetes and their families. You might consider appropriateness for the child with diabetes, as well as the parents and/or siblings. You may do a search and select your own websites or choose from the following established sites:
   - www.diabetes.org
   - www.idcdiabetes.org
   - www.jdrf.org
   - www.niddk.nih.gov

Copyright © 2007 by Saunders, an imprint of Elsevier Inc. All rights reserved.

3. Discuss how you could suggest involving George Gonzalez's school nurse in his care.

4. Discuss strategies for dealing with the power struggles George and his mother seem to be having.

5. Do you think that George Gonzalez is a candidate for an insulin pump? Why or why not? Are there any ethical issues involved in your answer?

At this point, you have developed a basic understanding of diabetes in the school-age child. This understanding includes changing needs that occur with growth and development. Proceed to the next lesson for more on the application of teaching-learning principles in managing the problems of diabetes.

Copyright © 2007 by Saunders, an imprint of Elsevier Inc. All rights reserved.

LESSON 10

Teaching Self-Care to a Child with Diabetes and His Family

∽ **Reading Assignment:** The Child with an Endocrine or Metabolic Alteration
(Chapter 27, pages 898-915)

Patient: George Gonzalez, Room 301

Objectives:

- Identify learning needs of a child newly diagnosed with diabetes.
- Develop a sequential plan for teaching a child self-care of diabetes.
- Discuss approaches to teaching various information and skills based on level of growth and development.
- Explore need for information, readiness, capability, and motivation as significant factors in the teaching-learning process for working with parents and children with diabetes mellitus.
- Differentiate roles of the child and the parent in managing the child's diabetes.

In this lesson you will be focusing on the teaching aspect of the care of a child with diabetes. You will consider learning needs according to developmental stage and parental responsibilities, along with the dynamic nature of supervision and self-care. You may need to review developmental issues associated with various age groups. You may also need to review the teaching-learning process since you will be applying principles throughout your work. You will assess needs, capabilities, readiness, and motivation. As you plan care, you will move beyond "teach about . . ." interventions and will begin more carefully articulating both the content (the "information or skill") to be taught and the method (the "how") to be used.

Copyright © 2007 by Saunders, an imprint of Elsevier Inc. All rights reserved.

Exercise 1

Clinical Preparation: Writing Activity

30 minutes

1. Review the information in the box on pages 909-910 in your textbook. How will you determine the learning needs of a child with diabetes and his family? What are your general thoughts about the influence of different developmental stages? (*Hint:* You do not need to break this task down into age groups.) What is the role and responsibility of the family in care?

2. What are some care issues if the child with diabetes is a toddler? What might you suggest to parents?

3. What are some care issues if the child with diabetes is a preschooler? What might you suggest to parents?

Copyright © 2007 by Saunders, an imprint of Elsevier Inc. All rights reserved.

4. What are some care issues if the child with diabetes is school-age? What might you suggest to parents?

5. What are some care issues if the child with diabetes is an adolescent? What might you suggest to parents?

6. Discuss general areas of content that you would want to include about diabetes when teaching a family.

7. Did you consider the "honeymoon phase" as part of your discussion? Why is this significant to parent teaching? What about this phase should you discuss with parents?

Copyright © 2007 by Saunders, an imprint of Elsevier Inc. All rights reserved.

Exercise 2

 CD-ROM Activity

30 minutes

- Sign in to work at Pacific View Regional Hospital for Period of Care 1. (*Note:* If you are already in the virtual hospital from a previous exercise, click on **Leave the Floor** and then **Restart the Program** to get to the sign-in window.)
- From the Patient List, select George Gonzalez (Room 301).
- Click on **Go to Nurses' Station** and then on **301**.
- Click on **Patient Care** and then on **Nurse-Client Interactions**.
- Select and view the video titled **0730: Supervision—Glucose Testing**. (*Note:* Check the virtual clock to see whether enough time has elapsed. You can use the fast-forward feature to advance the time by 2-minute intervals if the video is not yet available. Then click again on **Patient Care** and **Nurse-Client Interactions** to refresh the screen.)

1. Is George Gonzalez physically capable of being responsible for his own blood glucose testing?

2. What are some reasons why George Gonzalez may be noncompliant with blood glucose testing?

3. What does the nurse do that is effective? What other interventions can be offered?

Copyright © 2007 by Saunders, an imprint of Elsevier Inc. All rights reserved.

4. Complete the chart below on teaching about insulin administration. For each aspect of teaching, fill in the appropriate content to discuss and method(s) for teaching about the content. The first row has been completed for you.

Aspect of Teaching	Content	Method(s)
Insulin	Characteristics and storage	Explanation, demonstration of appearance of different types, practice with reading different labels
Syringes and preparing dose		
Injection		

5. Discuss the rationale for using a variety of methods for teaching insulin administration. Incorporate into your discussion how you would keep a family from becoming discouraged.

6. What are possible barriers to learning the skill of injection technique?

Copyright © 2007 by Saunders, an imprint of Elsevier Inc. All rights reserved.

7. List areas of content to address when discussing site rotations.

8. What is the site from which insulin is most rapidly absorbed?

9. Develop a creative strategy for assisting with site rotations.

Exercise 3

 CD-ROM Activity

 30 minutes

- Sign in to work at Pacific View Regional Hospital on the Pediatrics Floor for Period of Care 2. (*Note:* If you are already in the virtual hospital from a previous exercise, click on **Leave the Floor** and then **Restart the Program** to get to the sign-in window.)
- From the Patient List, select George Gonzalez (Room 301).
- Click on **Go to Nurses' Station** and then on **301**.
- Click on **Patient Care** and then on **Nurse-Client Interactions**.
- Select and view the video titled **1115: Teaching—Disease Process**. (*Note:* Check the virtual clock to see whether enough time has elapsed. You can use the fast-forward feature to advance the time by 2-minute intervals if the video is not yet available. Then click again on **Patient Care** and **Nurse-Client Interactions** to refresh the screen.)

1. Evaluate George Gonzalez's understanding of his condition and management of hypo-glycemia.

Copyright © 2007 by Saunders, an imprint of Elsevier Inc. All rights reserved.

2. What is his mother's level of understanding?

3. Given the responses of George Gonzalez and his mother, is there a need for teaching in this area? If so, what is the need?

 • Click on **Leave the Floor** and then **Restart the Program**.
 • Sign in to work at Pacific View Regional Hospital for Period of Care 3.
 • From the Patient List, select George Gonzalez (Room 301).
 • Click on **Go to Nurses' Station** and then on **301**.
 • Click on **Patient Care** and then on **Nurse-Client Interactions**.
 • Select and view the video titled **1500: Teaching—Diabetic Diet**. (*Note:* Check the virtual clock to see whether enough time has elapsed. You can use the fast-forward feature to advance the time by 2-minute intervals if the video is not yet available. Then click again on **Patient Care** and **Nurse-Client Interactions** to refresh the screen.)

4. What is George's diet order? What are the recommendations of the dietitian?

5. What is the current thinking as to dietary recommendations for the child with diabetes?

Copyright © 2007 by Saunders, an imprint of Elsevier Inc. All rights reserved.

6. Evaluate the nurse's teaching during the interaction. In regard to diet, what did she do well? What could she have done better?

7. Discuss the effects of physical activity on blood glucose. Consider times of day when George might have more activity than others. What should he do to prevent any activity-related problems?

8. Based on the potential complications discussed in question 7, do you think it would be better if George Gonzalez did not exercise? Explain your response. (*Hint:* Be sure to consider growth and development as a factor.)

Copyright © 2007 by Saunders, an imprint of Elsevier Inc. All rights reserved.

Exercise 4

Clinical Preparation: Writing Activity

15 minutes

1. Health maintenance and regular visits with health care providers are important, even when the child is doing well. Discuss the issue of who (parent, child, or both) should be in attendance at an office visit.

2. What barriers do you see to providing optimal outpatient care for the child with diabetes and the family?

3. Discuss the advantages of diabetes groups or camps for a child like George Gonzalez.

Copyright © 2007 by Saunders, an imprint of Elsevier Inc. All rights reserved.

LESSON **11**

The Hospitalized Adolescent

/👓 **Reading Assignment:** Health Promotion for the Adolescent (Chapter 8, pages 185-205)
The Ill Child in the Hospital and Other Care Settings
(Chapter 11, pages 285-289, 292-293)

Patient: Tiffany Sheldon, Room 305

Objectives:

- Discuss growth and development tasks for the adolescent.
- Discuss how adolescent development affects approaches to nursing care.
- Identify stressors common to the hospitalized adolescent.
- Develop strategies to minimize the effect of stressors for the hospitalized adolescent.

In this lesson you will learn about some of the many challenges associated with the care of adolescents in the hospital setting. One thing that will become evident is the push and pull between childhood and adulthood, as well as the push and pull between the teen and her parents.

Exercise 1

✏️ **Clinical Preparation: Writing Activity**

 30 minutes

1. What are the major physical changes that occur in adolescence?

Copyright © 2007 by Saunders, an imprint of Elsevier Inc. All rights reserved.

2. Explain Tanner staging and discuss its significance for nurses.

3. Identify and explain Erikson's task for psychosocial development for the teen years.

4. Discuss the role of the peer group in regard to psychosocial development.

5. What is Piaget's task for adolescence?

Copyright © 2007 by Saunders, an imprint of Elsevier Inc. All rights reserved.

6. Adolescent behaviors can be broken down into early, middle, and late characteristics. Match each adolescent behavior below with the stage of adolescence in which the behavior is most likely to occur. This will be helpful in assisting you to think in terms of developmental sequence.

Adolescent Behavior	**Stage of Adolescence**
_____ Intense body image concerns	a. Early adolescence
_____ Emphasis on conformity	b. Middle adolescence
_____ Same-sex relationships	c. Late adolescence
_____ Abstract thinking	
_____ Increased self-esteem	
_____ Hanging out at the mall	
_____ Being impulsive and impatient	
_____ Feeling more secure with limits and discipline	
_____ Clashing with others over values	
_____ Having interest in the opposite sex	
_____ Rebelliousness	
_____ Telling personal fables	
_____ Setting career goals	
_____ Conceptualizing verbally	
_____ Becoming more introspective	
_____ Relationships becoming more mature	
_____ Daydreaming and fantasizing about glamorous roles	
_____ Having a part-time job	
_____ Having lasting friendships	

Copyright © 2007 by Saunders, an imprint of Elsevier Inc. All rights reserved.

7. Discuss the developmental issues in a teen's life that could contribute to one of the following: risk for pregnancy, risk for substance abuse, risk for alcohol abuse, or risk for smoking.

8. For the issue(s) you identified in question 7, what are some primary prevention strategies the nurse can use? Set your own nursing role: hospital nurse, school nurse, office nurse, etc.

Exercise 2

 CD-ROM Activity

 30 minutes

• Sign in to work at Pacific View Regional Hospital for Period of Care 1. (*Note:* If you are already in the virtual hospital from a previous exercise, click on **Leave the Floor** and then **Restart the Program** to get to the sign-in window.
• From the Patient List, select Tiffany Sheldon (Room 305).
• Click on **Go to Nurses' Station**.
• Click on **Chart** and then on **305**.
• Click on and review the **History and Physical** and **Emergency Department** tabs.

 1. What in Tiffany Sheldon's records is consistent with *Healthy People 2010* Objectives for Adolescents? (*Hint:* See page 186 in your textbook.)

Copyright © 2007 by Saunders, an imprint of Elsevier Inc. All rights reserved.

2. Provide some examples in Tiffany's chart that are indicative of her progress with cognitive development.

➡ • Click on **Return to Nurses' Station** and then on **305**.
   • Click on **Patient Care** and then on **Physical Assessment**.
   • Complete a head-to-toe assessment.

3. Using Tanner's stages for sexual maturity, identify the stage of Tiffany's sexual development.

4. What evidence shows that Tiffany Sheldon is undernourished?

5. What are some of the stressors of hospitalization for an adolescent?

6. Select one stressor that you identified above and determine some strategies to facilitate coping. Incorporate Tiffany's specific situation into your discussion.

Copyright © 2007 by Saunders, an imprint of Elsevier Inc. All rights reserved.

Exercise 3

Clinical Preparation: Writing Activity

30 minutes

1. List some words related to sexuality with which the nurse must be comfortable in order to talk with teens about sexual issues. Say these words out loud.

2. Choose one of the words that you identified in question 1 and list as many slang terms for the word as possible. Again, say the words out loud. Consider the reasons that you think you are being asked this question.

3. If your teenage patient says, "My boyfriend may have given me a disease, but you can't tell my parents," how would you respond? (*Hint:* There are two parts to this question.)

4. If Tiffany Sheldon, who is 14 years old, had a positive pregnancy test, what feelings would you have about working with her and her mother?

Copyright © 2007 by Saunders, an imprint of Elsevier Inc. All rights reserved.

5. How might Tiffany Sheldon's level of growth and development affect her response to her pregnancy?

6. If Tiffany Sheldon were pregnant, what would her options be? Reflect on your ability to "be present" and talk about any option she chooses.

7. Assume that Tiffany Sheldon has just said to you, "I have something to tell you, but you have to promise not to tell my mom." You feel you have a therapeutic relationship with Tiffany, and you are admittedly pleased that she feels so comfortable with you. But now you have to decide what to do. Select the most appropriate response from the following choices.
   a. "Of course I will promise. You can tell me anything."
   b. "I want to talk with you, but I can't promise to keep a secret if there is a concern about your safety."
   c. "Please don't tell me. You need to talk with your mother."
   d. "Everything has to be shared with a patient's parent. I will have to tell your mom what is going on."

8. What other nursing interventions might you carry out in this situation?

Copyright © 2007 by Saunders, an imprint of Elsevier Inc. All rights reserved.

12

Caring for a Teen with an Eating Disorder: Part 1

Reading Assignment: The Child with a Psychosocial Disorder
(Chapter 29, pages 971-975)

Patient: Tiffany Sheldon, Room 305

Objectives:

- Compare and contrast the descriptions, etiology, and typical behaviors associated with anorexia nervosa and bulimia nervosa.
- Discuss the physiologic impact of anorexia nervosa and bulimia nervosa.
- Discuss the developmental factors that put teens at risk for eating disorders.
- Discuss the multidisciplinary approach necessary for treatment of eating disorders.
- Explore the challenges of providing nursing care for patients with anorexia nervosa or bulimia nervosa.

In this lesson you will explore a variety of challenges associated with caring for a teen with an eating disorder. You will care for Tiffany Sheldon, a 14-year-old with a history of 18 admissions within the past year for complications associated with anorexia nervosa. In the process, you will learn about the physiologic implications of having an eating disorder.

Copyright © 2007 by Saunders, an imprint of Elsevier Inc. All rights reserved.

Exercise 1

Clinical Preparation: Writing Activity

🕐 30 minutes

1. Compare and contrast anorexia and bulimia by matching each characteristic below with the eating disorder in which it occurs. (*Hint:* Although some characteristics may seem to overlap, they are usually associated more closely with one problem rather than the other. Choose the problem most closely associated with each characteristic.)

Characteristics	Eating Disorder
_____ Deliberate refusal of food to maintain body weight	a. Anorexia nervosa
_____ Recurrent episodes of binge eating and a sense of loss of control	b. Bulimia nervosa
_____ Misuse of laxatives and/or diuretics	
_____ Amenorrhea	
_____ Overconcern with body image, though not distorted	
_____ Body image that is contrary to reality	
_____ Ritualistic eating pattern	
_____ Binge eating and purging	
_____ Muscle wasting, dull and brittle hair, lanugo	
_____ Electrolyte imbalance	
_____ Tooth erosion	
_____ Self-induced vomiting	
_____ Participation in sports, dance, or gymnastics is a risk factor	
_____ Cardiac arrhythmias	
_____ Excessive exercise	

2. Give an example of an eating pattern that might be found in a person with anorexia nervosa. What often underlies such behavior?

Copyright © 2007 by Saunders, an imprint of Elsevier Inc. All rights reserved.

3. How might family function and culture play into the problem of eating disorders?

4. What are some secondary gains achieved through eating disorders? (*Hint:* Secondary gains are the patient's perceived benefits besides weight loss.)

5. What are some characteristics of adolescents that put them at higher risk for an eating disorder?

6. Parents sometimes say at diagnosis that they had no idea that their child had a problem with an eating disorder. Why do you think this occurs?

Copyright © 2007 by Saunders, an imprint of Elsevier Inc. All rights reserved.

Exercise 2

 CD-ROM Activity

 30 minutes

- Sign in to work at Pacific View Regional Hospital for Period of Care 1. (*Note:* If you are already in the virtual hospital from a previous exercise, click on **Leave the Floor** and then **Restart the Program** to get to the sign-in window.)
- From the Patient List, select Tiffany Sheldon (Room 305).
- Click on **Go to Nurses' Station**.
- Click on **Chart** and then on **305**.
- Click on and review the **Nursing Admission** and **History and Physical** tabs.

1. What in Tiffany Sheldon's history is indicative of her diagnosis of anorexia nervosa?

 2. How much does Tiffany Sheldon weigh? In what percentile does her weight fall? (*Hint:* Refer to the growth chart found on page 1043 of your textbook.)

 - Click on **Return to Nurses' Station** and then on **305**.
- Click on **Patient Care**.
- Complete a head-to-toe assessment, watching for data consistent with anorexia nervosa.

Copyright © 2007 by Saunders, an imprint of Elsevier Inc. All rights reserved.

3. As you complete your assessment, what stands out to you? The patient's physical appearance? The systemic problems? How does nutritional status affect the total patient?

4. Complete the following table by giving a rationale for each of the physician's orders listed.

Physician's Order	Rationale
Blood chemistry	
HCG	
Drug serology	
VDRL	
Urine specific gravity	
Cardiac monitor	
IV fluids	
KCl added to IV	
Orthostatic BP measurements	

Copyright © 2007 by Saunders, an imprint of Elsevier Inc. All rights reserved.

Exercise 3

  CD-ROM Activity

45 minutes

The first concern with a patient who has anorexia nervosa is to correct any metabolic imbalances. Keep this in mind as you work through this exercise.

- Sign in to work at Pacific View Regional Hospital for Period of Care 1. (*Note:* If you are already in the virtual hospital from a previous exercise, click on **Leave the Floor** and then **Restart the Program** to get to the sign-in window.)
- From the Patient List, select Tiffany Sheldon (Room 305).
- Click on **Go to Nurses' Station**.
- Click on **Chart** and then on **305**.
- Click on and review the **Physician's Orders** and **Laboratory Reports** tabs.

1. What is being done to assess and manage Tiffany's fluid and electrolyte imbalance?

2. What do Tiffany's lab results tell you about her fluid and electrolyte status? Report on the ones that give you specific information.

3. Tiffany Sheldon did not have a pH level done. A patient with anorexia nervosa is at risk for metabolic acidosis. What would happen to the pH in this instance?

 - Click on **Return to Nurses' Station** and then on **305**.
- Click on **Patient Care** and then on **Physical Assessment**.
- Complete a head-to-toe assessment.

Copyright © 2007 by Saunders, an imprint of Elsevier Inc. All rights reserved.

4. List the objective assessment data that indicate dehydration.

5. Why is Tiffany on a cardiac monitor?

6. Tiffany is receiving IV fluid with potassium chloride added. What is the physician's order for this drug? What are the nursing responsibilities before and during potassium administration?

7. Complete the following steps to develop the priority nursing diagnosis for Tiffany Sheldon and identify related nursing interventions.

   a. Identify a generic nursing diagnosis for hydration problems in patients with anorexia nervosa.

Copyright © 2007 by Saunders, an imprint of Elsevier Inc. All rights reserved.

   b. Now rewrite this nursing diagnosis so that it accurately reflects Tiffany Sheldon's situation.

   c. Develop outcomes for this nursing diagnosis.

   d. Develop nursing interventions appropriate for meeting these outcomes.

You have explored the first phase of treatment for an eating disorder. Now proceed to the next lesson to learn about weight gain and the underlying psychosocial issues.

Copyright © 2007 by Saunders, an imprint of Elsevier Inc. All rights reserved.

Caring for a Teen with an Eating Disorder: Part 2

Reading Assignment: The Child with a Psychosocial Disorder
(Chapter 29, pages 971-975)

Patient: Tiffany Sheldon, Room 305

Objectives:

- Compare and contrast the descriptions, etiology, and typical behaviors associated with anorexia nervosa and bulimia nervosa.
- Discuss the physiologic impact of anorexia nervosa and bulimia nervosa.
- Discuss the developmental factors that put teens at risk for eating disorders.
- Discuss the multidisciplinary approach necessary for treatment of eating disorders.
- Explore the challenges of providing nursing care for patients with anorexia nervosa or bulimia nervosa.

You considered some of the physiologic implications of eating disorders in the previous lesson. Now you will explore how weight gain is accomplished and the psychiatric therapy that is necessary to prevent future recurrences of the disease.

Copyright © 2007 by Saunders, an imprint of Elsevier Inc. All rights reserved.

Exercise 1

 CD-ROM Activity

30 minutes

- Sign in to work at Pacific View Regional Hospital for Period of Care 1. (*Note:* If you are already in the virtual hospital from a previous exercise, click on **Leave the Floor** and then **Restart the Program** to get to the sign-in window.)
- From the Patient List, select Tiffany Sheldon (Room 305).
- Click on **Go to Nurses' Station**.
- Click on **Chart** and then on **305**.
- Click on and review the **Nursing Admission** and **History and Physical** tabs.

1. As you review Tiffany's chart, what is your reaction to her problem? Do you see her as having control over her situation? Is there a parenting concern evident?

2. Brainstorm a list of areas of concern that haven't been mentioned that you would like to explore further.

Copyright © 2007 by Saunders, an imprint of Elsevier Inc. All rights reserved.

3. What in Tiffany's history is indicative of her diagnosis of anorexia nervosa? (*Hint:* You may refer to your response to Exercise 2, question 1 in the previous lesson.)

4. Did you identify family crisis (divorce of parents) as a possible precipitating factor in Tiffany's situation? Did you include the fact that she is an "A" student on your list? Why should you see these factors as red flags?

→ • Click on **Return to Nurses' Station** and then on **305**.
  • Click on **Patient Care** and then on **Nurse-Client Interactions**.
  • Select and view the video titled **0730: Initial Assessment**. (*Note:* Check the virtual clock to see whether enough time has elapsed. You can use the fast-forward feature to advance the time by 2-minute intervals if the video is not yet available. Then click again on **Patient Care** and **Nurse-Client Interactions** to refresh the screen.)

Copyright © 2007 by Saunders, an imprint of Elsevier Inc. All rights reserved.

5. Tiffany Sheldon has been described as having a flat affect, being withdrawn, and avoiding eye contact. How would you describe her behavior at the time of this interaction?

6. What is the most effective communication to use with Tiffany Sheldon?

7. Suppose Tiffany tells you that she is fat. How would you respond? Put your response in the actual words you would use.

8. What is the relationship between body image, need for control, and Tiffany Sheldon's eating disorder?

Copyright © 2007 by Saunders, an imprint of Elsevier Inc. All rights reserved.

9. You have already looked at the first phase of treatment: medical correction of electrolyte imbalance and monitoring the effects (especially cardiac). What other multidimensional interventions are important for Tiffany Sheldon?

10. How do you think Tiffany might respond to being told that she will be seen by an Eating Disorders Team?

11. What is the nurse's role in identifying and/or coordinating care and services that Tiffany requires during her inpatient stay?

Exercise 2

 CD-ROM Activity

 45 minutes

Now, begin thinking about how adequate caloric intake is achieved.

- Sign in to work at Pacific View Regional Hospital for Period of Care 2. (*Note:* If you are already in the virtual hospital from a previous exercise, click on **Leave the Floor** and then **Restart the Program** to get to the sign-in window.)
- From the Patient List, select Tiffany Sheldon (Room 305).
- Click on **Go to Nurses' Station** and then on **305**.
- Click on **Patient Care** and then on **Nurse-Client Interactions**.
- Select and view the video titled **1115: Managing Anorexia Nervosa**. (*Note:* Check the virtual clock to see whether enough time has elapsed. You can use the fast-forward feature to advance the time by 2-minute intervals if the video is not yet available. Then click again on **Patient Care** and **Nurse-Client Interactions** to refresh the screen.)

Copyright © 2007 by Saunders, an imprint of Elsevier Inc. All rights reserved.

1. Discuss the cultural beliefs and personal perceptions that might influence the development of an eating disorder in a teen.

2. What is the value of an eating contract for Tiffany Sheldon?

→ • Click on **Chart** and then on **305**.
  • Click on and review the **Physician's Orders** for diet orders.
  • Click on Return to Room **305**.
  • Click on **Patient Care** and then on **Nurse-Client Interactions**.
  • Select and view the video titled **1130: Monitoring Compliance**. (*Note:* Check the virtual clock to see whether enough time has elapsed. You can use the fast-forward feature to advance the time by 2-minute intervals if the video is not yet available. Then click again on **Patient Care** and **Nurse-Client Interactions** to refresh the screen.)

3. What is the rationale for the diet orders as part of the eating contract?

4. Calculate Tiffany Sheldon's daily caloric needs.

5. What supportive interventions might the nurse provide to help Tiffany remain compliant?

Copyright © 2007 by Saunders, an imprint of Elsevier Inc. All rights reserved.

Now consider the emotional aspects of Tiffany Sheldon's care.

- Click on **Leave the Floor** and then **Restart the Program**.
- Sign in to work at Pacific View Regional Hospital for Period of Care 3.
- From the Patient List, select Tiffany Sheldon (Room 305).
- Click on **Go to Nurses' Station** and then on **305**.
- Click on **Patient Care** and then on **Nurse-Client Interactions**.
- Select and view the video titled **1500: Relapse—Contributing Factors**. (*Note:* Check the virtual clock to see whether enough time has elapsed. You can use the fast-forward feature to advance the time by 2-minute intervals if the video is not yet available. Then click again on **Patient Care** and **Nurse-Client Interactions** to refresh the screen.)

6. What does Tiffany say has caused her relapse? What recent events, if any, may have contributed to an acute episode of her anorexia nervosa?

7. What did the psychiatrist do to effectively elicit Tiffany's concerns?

- Click on **Patient Care** and then on **Nurse-Client Interactions**.
- Select and view the video titled **1530: Facilitating Success**. (*Note:* Check the virtual clock to see whether enough time has elapsed. You can use the fast-forward feature to advance the time by 2-minute intervals if the video is not yet available. Then click again on **Patient Care** and **Nurse-Client Interactions** to refresh the screen.)

8. What multidimensional factors will contribute to Tiffany's ability to comply with the eating contract? What barriers may be present?

Copyright © 2007 by Saunders, an imprint of Elsevier Inc. All rights reserved.

9. A patient with an eating disorder may not like the sensations associated with refeeding. Develop strategies to help Tiffany overcome barriers to the success of her eating disorder plan.

Exercise 3

Clinical Preparation: Writing Activity

15 minutes

1. Lets assume that Tiffany Sheldon refuses to eat and that her condition puts her at greater health risk. The hospital is awaiting a court order for a feeding tube. Tiffany will need to be restrained if the order is implemented. How will you handle this situation? What are your responsibilities as a nurse?

Copyright © 2007 by Saunders, an imprint of Elsevier Inc. All rights reserved.

2. Nurses in community settings may play several roles with teens who have anorexia nervosa, one of which is case finding. Discuss this role.

3. If you are working in a community setting and a teen said to you, "I have to tell you something, but you have to promise not to tell anyone," how would you respond? What would your responsibilities be?

Generally, when the facilities are available, patients with eating disorders are transferred to an Eating Disorders Unit where professionals are highly skilled and experienced with care. However, this may not be the case in all settings. Thus all nurses need to be aware of the problems, risks, and usual approaches to treatment. You have accomplished this by completing this lesson.

Copyright © 2007 by Saunders, an imprint of Elsevier Inc. All rights reserved.

LESSON **14**

Caring for a Child and Family in the Emergency Department

/𝒪𝒪 **Reading Assignment:** Emergency Care of the Child (Chapter 10, pages 250-269)
The Child with a Neurologic Alteration
(Chapter 28, pages 923-931, 942-945)

Patient: Tommy Douglas, Room 302

Objectives:

- Identify factors that may culminate in a stressful environment in the Emergency Department (ED).
- Discuss nursing interventions supportive of the child and family who are in the ED.
- Discuss the concept of "across the room" assessment and priority setting for a child in the ED.
- Explore the implications of growth and development in emergency care.
- Explore medications frequently used in traumatic emergency situations.

In this lesson you will explore the role of the nurse in Emergency department care. More often than not, the priority needs of the child will be physiologic, but the psychosocial element of care cannot be ignored. Parents have many support needs that sometimes are pushed aside during the acute phase of the visit. You will learn general strategies for dealing with such issues. You will be working with 6-year-old Tommy Douglas, who arrived in the Emergency Department after a blunt trauma injury.

Copyright © 2007 by Saunders, an imprint of Elsevier Inc. All rights reserved.

Exercise 1

Clinical Preparation: Writing Activity

30 minutes

1. List and explain five or six factors that can contribute to creating a stressful environment when a child is brought to the Emergency Department after a traumatic event.

2. Did you include growth and development on your list? Give an example of how it would make a difference in your care.

3. For each of the factors you listed in question 1, develop a nursing intervention to minimize stress. If you have had experience in such an environment (even during an observation), you have an opportunity to be creative here.

Copyright © 2007 by Saunders, an imprint of Elsevier Inc. All rights reserved.

4. Review the general guidelines for minimizing stress on page 254 of your textbook. How many of them did you incorporate in your intervention list? For any interventions you listed that are not in the textbook, consider how easy or realistic they would be to implement. Write a reflective comment.

5. What is meant by the notion of "assessment from across the room"? Identify some assessments that can be made in this manner.

6. Identify the priority assessment for any child brought to the Emergency Department.

7. Rank the following care items in order of priority by numbering from 1 (highest priority) to 7 (lowest priority).

Care Item	Priority Ranking
Trauma scoring	
Assessment of child's coping	
Circulatory assessment	
History of injury	
Breathing assessment	
Airway assessment	
Signs of other injury	

Copyright © 2007 by Saunders, an imprint of Elsevier Inc. All rights reserved.

8. Choose two age groups of children that you would find especially challenging to work with in the Emergency Department. For each age group, explain the challenges and share a nursing intervention to help.

Parents and caregivers need a great deal of support. Nurses need to be able to anticipate fears and anxieties in order to craft careful communication to elicit and respond to concerns.

9. What are the three greatest fears parents have when their child is brought to the Emergency Department?

10. Parents may feel pushed aside in the ED. How can the nurse deal with this problem?

Copyright © 2007 by Saunders, an imprint of Elsevier Inc. All rights reserved.

Exercise 2

 CD-ROM Activity

 45 minutes

- Sign in to work at Pacific View Regional Hospital for Period of Care 1. (*Note:* If you are already in the virtual hospital from a previous exercise, click on **Leave the Floor** and then **Restart the Program** to get to the sign-in window.)
- From the Patient List, select Tommy Douglas (Room 302).
- Click on **Go to Nurses' Station**.
- Click on **Chart** and then on **302**.
- Click on and review the **Emergency Department** and **Physician's Orders** tabs.

1. Review the circumstances of Tommy Douglas' admission. Include such information as the nature of his injury and the people around him.

2. Tommy Douglas reportedly fell from a swing and hit his head on concrete. This is considered to be a blunt trauma injury. Explain what is meant by blunt trauma.

3. Review Tommy's initial medication orders (from admission on Tuesday through Wednesday morning). List each of the medications ordered and give a reason for each order.

 - Click on **Return to Nurses' Station**.
- Click on the **Drug** icon in the lower left corner of the screen.
- Review the medications ordered for Tommy Douglas, looking for any information you need to administer them safely and correctly.

Copyright © 2007 by Saunders, an imprint of Elsevier Inc. All rights reserved.

4. Do you have any concerns about the medications ordered? Explain.

→ Select one of the medications that needs to be administered during this period of care and complete the following steps to prepare and administer it.

- Click on **Return to Nurses' Station** and then on **Medication Room**.
- Using the Six Rights, select, prepare, and administer the medication to be given. When you have finished the preparation, return to Tommy Douglas' room and administer the medication. (*Hint:* Although you should be getting more comfortable with the steps of preparing and administering medications, you can refer to pages 26-30 and 37-41 in the **Getting Started** section if you need help.)
- To obtain feedback, click on **Leave the Floor**.
- Click on **Look at Your Preceptor's Evaluations** and then on **Medication Scorecard**.

5. Review the feedback on your Medication Scorecard. Are there any areas in which you need to make changes? If so, select another medication ordered for Tommy and practice the procedure again.

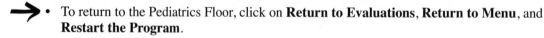

- To return to the Pediatrics Floor, click on **Return to Evaluations**, **Return to Menu**, and **Restart the Program**.
- Sign in to work at Pacific View Regional Hospital for Period of Care 1.
- From the Patient List, select Tommy Douglas (Room 302).
- Click on **Go to Nurses' Station**.
- Click on **Chart** and then on **302**.
- Click on and review the **Physician's Orders** tab.

6. $NaHCO_3$ is ordered to be given STAT. How much time do you have to prepare and administer the medication?

Copyright © 2007 by Saunders, an imprint of Elsevier Inc. All rights reserved.

7. Why is Tommy receiving bolus infusions?

 • Click on and review the **Nursing Admission** tab.

8. The physician has ordered a rate increase for norepinephrine. At what rate was the drug running, and to what rate has it been increased? (*Hint:* Find Tommy's weight in the Nursing Admission to do the necessary calculations.)

9. Tommy's blood pressure is low. Explain why fluids help to maintain blood pressure.

In this lesson, you have considered care for the family whose child has been brought to the Emergency Department. As a matter of priorities, you have undertaken a brief look at general assessment and medications commonly administered. Proceed to the next lesson for more specific exploration of care for a child with a head injury.

Copyright © 2007 by Saunders, an imprint of Elsevier Inc. All rights reserved.

15 ⎯⎯⎯⎯⎯⎯⎯⎯⎯⎯⎯⎯⎯⎯⎯⎯⎯⎯⎯

Emergency Care for a Child with a Head Injury

⎯⎯⎯

Reading Assignment: The Child with a Neurologic Alteration
(Chapter 28, pages 923-931, 942-945)

Patient: Tommy Douglas, Room 302

Objectives:

- Differentiate among various types of head injuries.
- Identify priority concerns related to head injury.
- Discuss the use of the Glasgow Coma Scale in children.
- Discuss support for parents of a child who has suffered a head injury.

In this lesson you will learn about the care of a child with a head injury and the various types of head injuries and associated problems. You will work with 6-year-old Tommy Douglas who has arrived in the Emergency Department after a blunt trauma injury.

Exercise 1

Clinical Preparation: Writing Activity

45 minutes

If you have completed Lesson 14, you are familiar with the basics of initial care of a child with a traumatic injury who is in the ED. Now you will focus more specifically on head injuries.

1. What is the leading cause of death in children?

2. What is unique about school-age children with regard to unintentional injuries?

Copyright © 2007 by Saunders, an imprint of Elsevier Inc. All rights reserved.

3. Identify common causes of head injuries in children.

4. List and define the types of head injuries.

5. Based on the list you just completed, what are some nursing concerns?

Copyright © 2007 by Saunders, an imprint of Elsevier Inc. All rights reserved.

6. Explain the mechanism of the acceleration-deceleration injury that occurs with a major head injury.

7. What are the priorities for initial management of a head injury?

8. A child with a head injury is at risk for _____

   and _____.

9. List the signs of increased intracranial pressure.

10. Identify and differentiate between the two general types of seizures.

11. Which type of seizure activity is more likely to be observed in a child with a head injury?

Copyright © 2007 by Saunders, an imprint of Elsevier Inc. All rights reserved.

12. Describe the Glasgow Coma Scale (GCS). Include the parameters that are assessed when it is used, particularly in children. (*Hint:* Review adaptations for children on page 928 of your textbook.)

Exercise 2

CD-ROM Activity

45 minutes

- Sign in to work at Pacific View Regional Hospital for Period of Care 1. (*Note:* If you are already in the virtual hospital from a previous exercise, click on **Leave the Floor** and then **Restart the Program** to get to the sign-in window.)
- From the Patient List, select Tommy Douglas (Room 302).
- Click on **Go to Nurses' Station**.
- Click on **Chart** and then on **302**.
- Click on and review the **Emergency Department** and **Physician's Orders** tabs.

1. Review the circumstances of Tommy Douglas' admission. Include information such as the nature of his injury and the people around him.

2. What significant neurologic data did you find in Tommy Douglas' ED record?

Copyright © 2007 by Saunders, an imprint of Elsevier Inc. All rights reserved.

3. Tommy Douglas is being stabilized in preparation for transfer to the Intensive Care Unit. A cerebral perfusion scan is done. What is the purpose of this test?

It is determined that Tommy Douglas will not be going to the Intensive Care Unit as planned. He is instead being transferred to the Pediatric Unit for end-of-life care.

4. Tommy's family is very fearful about his transfer. They don't want to leave the staff and believe that more is being done for him where he is. How would you respond?

 • Click on **Return to Nurses' Station** and then on **302**.

• Click on **Patient Care**.

• Complete a focused neurologic assessment of Tommy Douglas and then chart your findings in the EPR. (*Hint:* If you need help entering data in the EPR, refer to pages 15-16 in the **Getting Started** section of this workbook.)

• Click on **Leave the Floor** and then **Look at Your Preceptor's Evaluations**.

• Select **Examination Report** and review your evaluation.

5. Reflect on the completeness of your focused assessment of Tommy's neurologic status.

Copyright © 2007 by Saunders, an imprint of Elsevier Inc. All rights reserved.

• Click on **Return to Evaluations**, **Return to Menu**, and **Restart the Program**.
- Sign in to work at Pacific View Regional Hospital for Period of Care 1.
- From the Patient List, select Tommy Douglas (Room 302).
- Click on **Go to Nurses' Station** and then on **302**.
- Click on **Patient Care** and then on **Nurse-Client Interactions**.
- Select and view the video titled **0730: Assessment—Neurological**. (*Note:* Check the virtual clock to see whether enough time has elapsed. You can use the fast-forward feature to advance the time by 2-minute intervals if the video is not yet available. Then click again on **Patient Care** and **Nurse-Client Interactions** to refresh the screen.)

6. What was Tommy's GCS score?

7. Reflect on how well the nurse explained the use and meaning of the GCS scoring. Do you think the parents found support during this interaction? What, if anything, would you have done differently?

 • Click on **Patient Care** and then on **Nurse-Client Interactions**.
- Select and view the video titled 0745: Intervention—Airway. (*Note:* Check the virtual clock to see whether enough time has elapsed. You can use the fast-forward feature to advance the time by 2-minute intervals if the video is not yet available. Then click again on **Patient Care** and **Nurse-Client Interactions** to refresh the screen.)

Copyright © 2007 by Saunders, an imprint of Elsevier Inc. All rights reserved.

8. Tommy Douglas is on a ventilator. What is a ventilator used for? How would you expect his ventilator to be set?

9. How would you explain to Tommy's parents what the ventilator is doing?

Tommy Douglas will be receiving end-of-life care. Continue to the next lesson to learn about effective nursing care for the parents and family of a child who is dying.

Copyright © 2007 by Saunders, an imprint of Elsevier Inc. All rights reserved.

Providing Support for Families Experiencing the Loss of a Child

 Reading Assignment: Foundations of Child Health Nursing (Chapter 1, pages 10-11)
The Child with a Chronic Condition or a Terminal Illness
(Chapter 12, pages 320-331)

Patient: Tommy Douglas, Room 302

Objectives:

- Explore the range of reactions that may occur when a family is told there is no hope of saving a child's life.
- Discuss the role of hospital ethics committees.
- Discuss nursing responsibilities associated with organ donation.
- Discuss the concept of "allowing" a child to die.
- Identify strategies to support parents and children as a child dies.

In this lesson you will explore circumstances that may occur in hospital settings around a traumatic event resulting in certainty of death. Care for parents and other family members is the major focus during this time of hospice care. You will continue to work with the family of 6-year-old Tommy Douglas as he dies.

Exercise 1

 CD-ROM Activity

45 minutes

- Sign in to work at Pacific View Regional Hospital for Period of Care 2. (*Note:* If you are already in the virtual hospital from a previous exercise, click on **Leave the Floor** and then **Restart the Program** to get to the sign-in window.)
- From the Patient List, select Tommy Douglas (Room 302).
- Click on **Go to Nurses' Station** and then on **302**.
- Click on **Patient Care** and then on **Nurse-Client Interactions**.
- Select and view the video titled **1115: The Family (Care) Conference**. (*Note:* Check the virtual clock to see whether enough time has elapsed. You can use the fast-forward feature to advance the time by 2-minute intervals if the video is not yet available. Then click again on **Patient Care** and **Nurse-Client Interactions** to refresh the screen.)

193

Copyright © 2007 by Saunders, an imprint of Elsevier Inc. All rights reserved.

1. Tommy Douglas has been certified as "brain dead," and a family conference has been held to inform his parents that he will not be helped by further intervention. Who are the usual participants in such a conference? What does each person bring to the discussion?

2. What is the role of the institutional ethics committee with respect to any potential conflicts in care delivery?

3. What intervention should the nurse provide to the parents after the family conference?

4. Assume that Tommy's family wants him to live "at all costs." How would you feel about this? What might be your response to Tommy's parents?

Copyright © 2007 by Saunders, an imprint of Elsevier Inc. All rights reserved.

• Click on **Patient Care** and then on **Nurse-Client Interactions**.
• Select and view the video titled **1130: Decision—Organ Donation**. (*Note:* Check the virtual clock to see whether enough time has elapsed. You can use the fast-forward feature to advance the time by 2-minute intervals if the video is not yet available. Then click again on **Patient Care** and **Nurse-Client Interactions** to refresh the screen.)

5. As Tommy's parents agree to organ donation, is there evidence of progression with anticipatory grieving?

6. Visit the website for United Network for Organ Sharing (www.unos.org). Discuss the criteria for donation and management of a potential donor.

 • Click on **Chart** and then on **302**.
• Click on and review the **Physician's Orders** tab.

7. Discuss the kind of care that is being provided for Tommy during this time.

8. Tommy is receiving hospice care. Contrast palliative care and hospice care.

Copyright © 2007 by Saunders, an imprint of Elsevier Inc. All rights reserved.

Let's check in on Tommy's family a little later in the day.

 • Click on **Leave the Floor** and then **Restart the Program**.
• Sign in to work at Pacific View Regional Hospital for Period of Care 3.
• From the Patient List, select Tommy Douglas (Room 302).
• Click on **Go to Nurses' Station** and then on **302**.
• Click on **Patient Care** and then on **Nurse-Client Interactions**.
• Select and view the video titled **1500: Nurse—Family Communication**. (*Note:* Check the virtual clock to see whether enough time has elapsed. You can use the fast-forward feature to advance the time by 2-minute intervals if the video is not yet available. Then click again on **Patient Care** and **Nurse-Client Interactions** to refresh the screen.)

9. Evaluate the nurse's approach in dealing with a family in crisis. Did the nurse demonstrate empathy? If so, how?

10. Is the nurse's body language congruent with his verbal communication?

11. Present an alternative to the nurse's approach if you believe it is indicated.

12. What if Tommy's parents ask to take him home. What would be your response?

Copyright © 2007 by Saunders, an imprint of Elsevier Inc. All rights reserved.

Exercise 2

Clinical Preparation: Writing Activity

45 minutes

"Allowing" a child to die is a very difficult concept. Parents go through several stages as their child dies.

1. Discuss what parents experience when their child experiences a life-threatening injury or illness that then becomes terminal.

2. Parents frequently need to talk about what is happening while their child is dying. Why?

3. What anticipatory guidance would you offer parents for dealing with the other children in their family?

4. What information needs to be provided about the dying process?

5. How might you guide parents at the time of death? (*Hint:* Remember that allowing a child to die is tremendously difficult for parents.)

Copyright © 2007 by Saunders, an imprint of Elsevier Inc. All rights reserved.

6. How are siblings of a dying child likely to view death?

7. How would you provide care for the family members after their child's death?

8. Assume that you enter the room and find the parents sobbing as they sit with their dying child. Does this mean you have not been effective with your teaching and care? What can you do for these parents?

9. What do you think the concept of "chronic sorrow" means?

Copyright © 2007 by Saunders, an imprint of Elsevier Inc. All rights reserved.

10. How do you think you might react to caring for a dying child and the family? Do you think you could be effective? Explain your response.

11. Discuss ways that nurses who care for dying children cope with their own grief.

You have had the opportunity to consider care of the terminally ill child and many of the issues that might arise. This experience will help you to be more effective with your nursing care in similar situations—and it will help you take better care of yourself.

Copyright © 2007 by Saunders, an imprint of Elsevier Inc. All rights reserved.

LESSON **17**

Safety for Infants and Young Children

🕶 **Reading Assignment:** Health Promotion for the Developing Child
(Chapter 4, pages 94-95)
Health Promotion for the Infant
(Chapter 5, pages 99, 122, 124-126, 128)
Health Promotion During Early Childhood
(Chapter 6, pages 137, 151-156)
Health Promotion for the School-Age Child
(Chapter 7, pages 165, 174-177)
Health Promotion for the Adolescent
(Chapter 8, pages 186, 199-200)

Patients: George Gonzalez, Room 301
Tommy Douglas, Room 302
Carrie Richards, Room 303
Stephanie Brown, Room 304
Tiffany Sheldon, Room 305

Objectives:

- Discuss safety concerns for infants, toddlers, preschoolers, school-age children, and adolescents.
- Identify areas of anticipatory guidance that relate to safety concerns in each age group.
- Discuss nursing interventions that relate to safety concerns in children.

In this lesson you will consider a variety of safety aspects for different age groups. The concept of safety will be considered from a broad perspective. You will learn how responsibility for safety progresses from parents being completely responsible for safety of infants and very young children, to shared responsibility as children grow, and finally to adolescents assuming full responsibility for their own safety.

Copyright © 2007 by Saunders, an imprint of Elsevier Inc. All rights reserved.

Exercise 1

Clinical Preparation: Writing Activity

 30 minutes

1. Review the *Healthy People 2010* objectives for each age group found in the boxes on pages 99, 137, 165, and 186 in your textbook. For each level of growth and development in the table below, identify the safety-related risks that apply. The section on infants has been completed for you as an example.

Level of Growth and Development	Safety-Related Risks
Infants	Poisoning
	Suffocation
	Unintentional injury
Toddlers and preschoolers	
School-age children	
Adolescents	

Copyright © 2007 by Saunders, an imprint of Elsevier Inc. All rights reserved.

2. Comment on your reactions to the scope of issues associated with safety. Consider why some of these issues occur and whether problems can be prevented.

3. Write a brief reaction paper on safety concerns for infancy through adolescence. Identify concerns and discuss the role nurses can play with regard to addressing the problem.

Reduction of Injuries and Deaths from Infancy Through Adolescence

Copyright © 2007 by Saunders, an imprint of Elsevier Inc. All rights reserved.

4. Explain the concept of anticipatory guidance as it relates to safety concerns.

Exercise 2

 CD-ROM Activity

 30 minutes

- Sign in to work at Pacific View Regional Hospital for Period of Care 3. (*Note:* If you are already in the virtual hospital from a previous exercise, click on **Leave the Floor** and then **Restart the Program** to get to the sign-in window.)
- From the Patient List, select Carrie Richards (Room 303).
- Click on **Go to Nurses' Station**.
- Click on **Chart** and then on **303**.
- Click on and review the **History and Physical** tab.

1. Using a very broad definition of safety, identify areas of concern where interventions need to be made regarding Carrie Richards' safety?

2. Identify one area of anticipatory guidance that would be appropriate for Carrie's mother. One example is that she will be able to roll over soon and safety implications must be addressed.

 - Click on and review the **Consultations** tab.

3. Identify one strength and one area of possible concern that may affect how well Carrie's mother can plan for and meet safety needs.

Copyright © 2007 by Saunders, an imprint of Elsevier Inc. All rights reserved.

Now let's look at safety for the toddler/preschool group.

 • Click on **Return to Nurses' Station**.
• Click on **Leave the Floor** and then **Restart the Program**.
• Sign in to work at Pacific View Regional Hospital for Period of Care 3.
• From the Patient List, select Stephanie Brown (Room 304).
• Click on **Go to Nurses' Station**.
• Click on **Chart** and then on **304**.
• Click on **History and Physical** and review.

4. Are there any safety concerns associated with Stephanie Brown's cerebral palsy? Provide evidence for your response.

5. What will you tell Stephanie's mother about promoting her child's physical growth and development while also being aware of safety concerns?

6. Stephanie Brown's mother says that Stephanie loves to play with the kitchen cupboards, pulling everything out and playing with the items. Should you talk to her about this type of play?

Copyright © 2007 by Saunders, an imprint of Elsevier Inc. All rights reserved.

7. Develop a plan for poisoning prevention for toddlers and preschoolers. Discuss factors in growth and development that put these children at risk for poisoning. Identify what parents should do to prevent poisoning in this age group and identify the nursing role in prevention. Discuss the role of the Emergency Department nurse when a poisoning event has occurred.

Poisoning Prevention Plan

Exercise 3

 CD-ROM Activity

 15 minutes

Now let's look at another age group and patient situation.

- Click on **Return to Nurses' Station**.
- Click on **Leave the Floor** and then **Restart the Program**.
- Sign in to work at Pacific View Regional Hospital for Period of Care 3.
- From the Patient List, select Tommy Douglas (Room 302).
- Click on **Go to Nurses' Station**.
- Click on **Chart** and then **302**.
- Click on and review the **History and Physical** tab.

1. Tommy Douglas' condition is critical; therefore this will not be an appropriate time for teaching about safety. For your learning purposes, though, discuss Tommy's injury and its cause.

Copyright © 2007 by Saunders, an imprint of Elsevier Inc. All rights reserved.

2. What is Tommy Douglas' age? Is playing on swings an appropriate activity for him?

3. What are the safety issues that need to be employed for this type of play?

4. Parents still have a great deal of responsibility for child safety at this age. Develop a teaching checklist for parents with regard to playground safety. What would you include?

5. Identify another safety concern for this age group. (*Hint:* You may want to review your response in Exercise 1, Question 1 of this lesson for ideas.)

Copyright © 2007 by Saunders, an imprint of Elsevier Inc. All rights reserved.

Exercise 4

 CD-ROM Activity

 30 minutes

Let's look at school-age safety considerations.

- Click on **Return to Nurses' Station**.
- Click on **Leave the Floor** and then **Restart the Program**.
- Sign in to work at Pacific View Regional Hospital for Period of Care 3.
- From the Patient List, select George Gonzalez (Room 301).
- Click on **Go to Nurses' Station**.
- Click on **Chart** and then on **301**.
- Click on and review the **History and Physical** tab.

1. Identify any safety risk factors in George Gonzalez's record.

2. George also needs to increase his level of exercise. How does this need relate to the safety problem identified in the previous question?

 • Click on **Return to Nurses' Station** and then on **301**.
- Click on **Patient Care** and then on **Nurse-Client Interactions**.
- Select and view the video titled **1500: Teaching—Diabetic Diet**. (*Note:* Check the virtual clock to see whether enough time has elapsed. You can use the fast-forward feature to advance the time by 2-minute intervals if the video is not yet available. Then click again on **Patient Care** and **Nurse-Client Interactions** to refresh the screen.)

3. Comment on the nurse's approach with diet teaching. What did she do well? What would you have done differently, if anything?

Copyright © 2007 by Saunders, an imprint of Elsevier Inc. All rights reserved.

4. As you are considering preventing and treating hypoglycemia as it relates to exercise, what would be your next step?

 • Click on **Patient Care** and then on **Nurse-Client Interactions**.
   • Select and view the video titled **1535: Teaching—Effects of Exercise**. (*Note:* Check the virtual clock to see whether enough time has elapsed. You can use the fast-forward feature to advance the time by 2-minute intervals if the video is not yet available. Then click again on **Patient Care** and **Nurse-Client Interactions** to refresh the screen.)

5. Discuss the elements that you would incorporate in a teaching plan on activity/exercise for George Gonzalez and his mother. Be specific about content and teaching method.

6. George Gonzalez says that he likes to ride his bicycle and will try to do that more. What safety information would you need to provide about bike safety?

 • Click on **Chart** and then on **301**.
   • Click on and review the **History and Physical** tab.

7. What is George Gonzalez's age and school grade level?

Copyright © 2007 by Saunders, an imprint of Elsevier Inc. All rights reserved.

8. What anticipatory guidance would you offer to George's mother with regard to physical growth and development while also being aware of safety concerns?

9. Provide an example of adolescent behavior that might affect George's safety.

10. Do you consider a child who is home alone after school at risk for injury? Explain your answer.

Exercise 5

 CD-ROM Activity

 15 minutes

Finally, let's move on to explore adolescent safety issues.

- Click on **Return to Room 301** and then on **Nurses' Station**.
- Click on **Leave the Floor** and then **Restart the Program**.
- Sign in to work at Pacific View Regional Hospital for Period of Care 3.
- From the Patient List, select Tiffany Sheldon (Room 305).
- Click on **Go to Nurses' Station**.
- Click on **Chart** and then on **305**.
- Click on and review the **History and Physical** tab.

Copyright © 2007 by Saunders, an imprint of Elsevier Inc. All rights reserved.

1. What safety risk factors do you note in Tiffany Sheldon's History and Physical?

➤ • Click on and review the **Physician's Orders** tab.

2. What orders are related to Tiffany Sheldon's age of 14 years?

3. Reducing the risk for suicide is a *Healthy People 2010* goal. How might you assess for suicide potential and plan treatment for the depressed individual?

4. Brainstorm and list several factors that may put teens at risk for injury.

Copyright © 2007 by Saunders, an imprint of Elsevier Inc. All rights reserved.

5. If you were a school nurse, what prevention strategies would you develop and implement?

6. Discuss the role of parents in regard to safety in teens. How involved do you think they should be?

You've explored safety across the years from infancy to adolescence. You've considered the role of the nurse in teaching with parents and with children. This lesson will help you with a variety of the vast number of topics applicable to preventing accidents and injury.

Copyright © 2007 by Saunders, an imprint of Elsevier Inc. All rights reserved.

LESSON 18

Medication Administration in Children

👓 **Reading Assignment:** Medicating Infants and Children (Chapter 14, pages 372-393)

Patients: George Gonzalez, Room 301
Tommy Douglas, Room 302
Carrie Richards, Room 303
Stephanie Brown, Room 304

Objectives:

- Discuss the physiology of children regarding its effect on medication administration.
- Discuss pediatric principles associated with medication administration.
- Practice calculating safe dosages for certain medications for selected patients.
- Consider growth and development in administering medications.
- Safely administer medications according to the Six Rights.

In this lesson you will review principles of medication administration in infants and children. You will also look at the impact of growth and development on the success of the medication administration experience and have the opportunity to administer medications in the virtual environment.

Exercise 1

✏️ **Clinical Preparation: Writing Activity**

 45 minutes

1. Explain the difference between pharmacokinetics and pharmacodynamics.

Copyright © 2007 by Saunders, an imprint of Elsevier Inc. All rights reserved.

2. Gastric acidity, gastric emptying time, GI motility, and function of pancreatic enzymes are four factors that influence absorption. How does the unique physiology of infants affect each of these factors? Record your answers in the table below.

Factor	Effect in Infants
Gastric acidity	
Gastric emptying time	
GI motility	
Function of pancreatic enzymes	

3. How do fluid volumes in children affect the distribution of medications differently than in adults?

4. Metabolism and excretion are important considerations. How does infant growth affect these?

Copyright © 2007 by Saunders, an imprint of Elsevier Inc. All rights reserved.

5. Review the section on psychologic and developmental factors found on pages 375-376 in your textbook. Identify one age group and create a clinical situation that requires application of these principles of medication administration.

6. Consider the following statement: It's possible for medication administration to become more difficult as the child gets better. Do you agree or disagree? Why?

7. Dosages are calculated based on a child's weight (mg/kg). What is another method for calculating safe dosages?

8. You have an order to administer ibuprofen 150 mg to a 2-year-old who weighs 22 pounds. The label on the bottle says 100 mg/5 mL. Calculate the dosage and decide whether the order is safe or not.

Copyright © 2007 by Saunders, an imprint of Elsevier Inc. All rights reserved.

9. Adherence to a full course of prescribed medication continues to be a problem. In the left column below, create a list of factors that might lead to lack of compliance. For each factor you list, identify a strategy that could be used to improve medication adherence.

Factors Affecting Compliance   **Interventions to Promote Compliance**

10. Identify whether each of the following statements regarding medication administration in children is true or false.

a. _____   If a decimal point is in the wrong place, there can be a 10-fold dosage error.

b. _____   It is acceptable practice to crush and mix medications with a serving of food.

c. _____   When using an oral syringe to give medication to an infant, squirt the medication along the side of the cheek.

d. _____   Otic medications should be administered with the pinna of the ear pulled up and back for a child under 3 years of age.

e. _____   Documentation of an injected medication includes the amount of the medication and the site used.

f. _____   The deltoid muscle is preferred over the vastus lateralis for intramuscular medications in young children.

g. _____   Asking "Do you want to take your medicine now?" is an effective approach to use with a toddler.

h. _____   It is acceptable practice for the parent to give an oral medication as long as the nurse takes responsibility for correct administration of the medication.

i. _____   To administer a rectal medication, position the child on the left side with the right leg flexed.

j. _____   Fluid administered IV is considered to be a medication.

Copyright © 2007 by Saunders, an imprint of Elsevier Inc. All rights reserved.

11. Some references present Five Rights and some present Six Rights for medication administration. List the Six Rights.

 12. EMLA cream can be used as a pharmacologic intervention to decrease pain and facilitate coping with injections or IV insertions. Review the Critical to Remember section found on page 387 of your textbook. What about this procedure is sometimes difficult to implement and therefore precludes the use of EMLA cream?

Exercise 2

 CD-ROM Activity

 60 minutes

- Sign in to work at Pacific View Regional Hospital for Period of Care 1. (*Note:* If you are already in the virtual hospital form a previous exercise, click on **Leave the Floor** and then **Restart the Program** to get to the sign-in window.)
- From the Patient List, select George Gonzalez (Room 301), Tommy Douglas (Room 302), Carrie Richards (Room 303), and Stephanie Brown (Room 304).
- Click on **Go to Nurses' Station**.
- Click on **MAR** and review medications that need to be administered at this time. Click on the tab with the individual room number for each patient whose MAR you need to review.

Copyright © 2007 by Saunders, an imprint of Elsevier Inc. All rights reserved.

1. Below, list the medications that need to be administered between 0700 and 0800 for each patient listed.

Patient	Medications Due Between 0700 and 0800
George Gonzalez	
Carrie Richards	
Stephanie Brown	
Tommy Douglas	

 • Click on **Return to Nurses' Station**.
  • Click on **Chart** and then select the room number of the first patient to whom you should give medication.
  • Within the chart, click on **Physician's Orders**.
  • Verify that the order and the MAR match. (*Note:* The Physician's Orders are the primary source of information. All other transfers of information need to be checked with the Physician's Orders.)

2. Which medication are you going to administer first and to whom? (*Note:* Tommy Douglas' medications are due at 0730 and 0800 and are part of treatments he is undergoing. They will be administered by the nurse caring for him. You are the nurse responsible for the rest of the medications.)

Copyright © 2007 by Saunders, an imprint of Elsevier Inc. All rights reserved.

3. George Gonzalez has 2 types of insulin ordered. What are they? Which is short-acting, and which is long-acting?

4. Is there a way of determining whether an insulin is short- or long-acting by looking at the medication in the vial? Explain.

5. You will be administering insulin in two separate doses. Most commonly, though, these insulins are mixed in one syringe. If administering in one syringe, which is drawn up first?

6. List the procedural steps for mixing insulins in one syringe.

7. Why is the procedure you outlined in question 6 used?

Copyright © 2007 by Saunders, an imprint of Elsevier Inc. All rights reserved.

Throughout the rest of this exercise, you will be instructed to administer medications to several of your patients. For each patient, follow the directions below:

- Click on **Go to Nurses' Station**.
- Click on the patient's room number to visit the patient.
- Click on **Take Vital Signs**.
- Click on **Clinical Alerts** and review the report.
- Click on **MAR** and find the order for the medication.
- Click on **Return to Room (Number)**.
- Click on **Medication Room**.
- Click on **Unit Dosage**.
- Click on drawer **(Room Number)**.
- Click on the drug desired.
- Click on **Put Medication on Tray**.
- Click on **Close Drawer**.
- Click on **View Medication Room**.
- Click on **Preparation**.
- Click on **Prepare** and follow the Preparation Wizard's prompts to complete preparation of the medication.
- Click on **Return to Medication Room**.
- Click on **Room Number** to return to the patient's room.
- Click on **Check Armband** and **Check Allergies**.
- Click on **Patient Care**.
- Click on **Medication Administration**.
- Find the medication listed on the left side of your screen. Click on the down arrow next to Select and choose **Administer**.
- Follow the Administration Wizard's prompts to administer the medication. Indicate Yes to document the administration in the MAR.
- Click on **Leave the Floor** and then **Look at Your Preceptor's Evaluations**.
- Click on **Medication Scorecard**.

8. Follow the steps listed above to prepare and administer George Gonzalez's insulin. How did you do? Reflect on your performance and consider anything you need to remember in the future in order to safely administer medications.

Copyright © 2007 by Saunders, an imprint of Elsevier Inc. All rights reserved.

9. You have several 0800 medications to administer. Start with Carrie Richards. What medication is ordered for her at this time? Will you be giving this medication? (*Note:* If you need to review the medication, you can use a nursing drug handbook or click on the **Drug** icon in the lower left corner of your screen.)

10. Move on to Stephanie Brown's medications. What medications are you going to administer at 0800?

11. Why are each of these drugs being used?

12. Prepare and administer Stephanie's medications (following the steps provided above question 8 in this exercise). Reflect on the experience and discuss areas of improvement and areas to work on.

As you walk by Carrie Richards' room, her mother says she would like her child to have some Tylenol and that she feels warm. You note that Carrie is sleeping quietly.

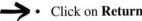
- Click on **Return to Nurses' Station**.
- Click on **Chart** and then on **303**.
- Click on and review the **Physician's Orders** tab.
- Click on **Return to Nurses' Station** and then on **MAR**.
- Check to verify that the MAR is correct.
- Click on **Return to Nurses' Station** and then on **303**.
- Check Carrie's temperature.

Copyright © 2007 by Saunders, an imprint of Elsevier Inc. All rights reserved.

13. Can Carrie have Tylenol for elevated temperature at this time?

14. When you next check Carrie's vital signs, her temperature is 100.8. She is also crying and fussy. Would you give her Tylenol at this time?

Following the steps provided above question 8 in this exercise, prepare and administer Tylenol to Carrie Richards.

15. What if the prn order for Tylenol read "for temp above 101 and irritability"? Legally, could you give Tylenol when Carrie Richards' temperature is at 101 degrees or below?

- Click on **Leave the Floor** and then **Restart the Program**.
- Sign in to work at Pacific View Regional Hospital for Period of Care 2.
- From the Patient List, select one or more of the patients.
- Again following the steps provided above question 8 of this exercise, prepare and administer several medications.
- Make sure at least one medication is an IV medication. (*Note:* The procedure is the same except the medications are found in the microinfusion bin rather than in the patient's drawer.)
- Continue on to Period of Care 3 to practice more medication administration.

16. In the space below, identify the medications you plan to administer and the use or action of each drug. Proceed through the procedure applying the Six Rights and administer the medications. Obtain your medication scorecard and reflect on the results.

You have undergone several practice experiences with administering medications. Though this process you have reinforced safe medication administration behavior. Congratulations!

Copyright © 2007 by Saunders, an imprint of Elsevier Inc. All rights reserved.

LESSON 19

Pediatric Nursing Care Management: Part 1

Reading Assignment: Review priorities of care for each of the following medical diagnoses and situations:
- Hospitalization of Children (Chapter 11, pages 288-304)
- Terminal Illness (Chapter 12, pages 320-331)
- Bronchiolitis (Chapter 21, pages 622-626)
- Diabetes Mellitus (Chapter 27, pages 898-915)
- Head Injury (Chapter 28, pages 927-931, 942-945)
- Cerebral Palsy (Chapter 28, pages 939-942)
- Meningitis (Chapter 28, pages 953-956)
- Anorexia Nervosa (Chapter 29, pages 971-975)
- Failure to Thrive (Chapter 29, pages 991-993)

Patients: George Gonzalez, Room 301
Tommy Douglas, Room 302
Carrie Richards, Room 303
Stephanie Brown, Room 304
Tiffany Sheldon, Room 305

Objectives:

- Set priorities in a given pediatric situation.
- Consider the nursing scope of practice for an RN and an LPN in making assignment decisions.
- Demonstrate the ability to make effective use of ancillary personnel.
- Demonstrate effective decision making in selected pediatric situations.
- Make room assignments for a group of pediatric patients.
- Develop a plan for care for a group of pediatric patients for the day.

In this lesson you will be asked to consider the roles and scope of practice of various health professionals and ancillary personnel. You will be applying principles of management and delegation as well as responding to events throughout a shift.

Copyright © 2007 by Saunders, an imprint of Elsevier Inc. All rights reserved.

Exercise 1

  CD-ROM Activity

60 minutes

- Sign in to work at Pacific View Regional Hospital for Period of Care 1. (*Note:* If you are already in the virtual hospital from a previous exercise, click on **Leave the Floor** and then **Restart the Program** to get to the sign-in window.)
- From the Patient List, select George Gonzalez (Room 301), Carrie Richards (Room 303), Stephanie Brown (Room 304), and Tiffany Sheldon (Room 305).
- Click on **Get Report** for George Gonzalez.
- After reading the report, click on **Return to Patient List**.
- Repeat the two previous steps for each of your assigned patients.

1. Assume that you and a nursing assistant are responsible for George Gonzalez, Carrie Richards, Stephanie Brown, and Tiffany Sheldon. Take notes on any concerns that you have and things that you need to do for each of these patients. Use two columns or create a system that will work for you as you provide care.

 - Click on **Go to Nurses' Station**.
- Click on **Chart** and then on **301**.
- Click on and review the **Physician's Orders** tab and add to your plan for the day.
- Repeat the two previous steps for each of your assigned patients.

Copyright © 2007 by Saunders, an imprint of Elsevier Inc. All rights reserved.

2. Identify the Physician's Orders that you need to address in your plan for the day.

3. Discuss aspects of care that you can safely assign to the nursing assistant and include your rationale.

4. Create a priority list of care responsibilities. Include who you will see first and the order in which you will visit each patient. Also include rationales for your decisions.

Copyright © 2007 by Saunders, an imprint of Elsevier Inc. All rights reserved.

5. The nurse is, of course, responsible for what the nursing assistant does. Discuss three of the tasks assigned to the nursing assistant and identify expectations that you would set.

Tasks Assigned	Expectations

Lets change the staffing mix for care of George Gonzalez, Carrie Richards, Stephanie Brown, and Tiffany Sheldon.

6. Assume that you are the charge nurse for the Pediatric Unit. You have four patients, and there is an LPN and a nursing assistant working with you. Having obtained report, determine how you will assign patient care. Complete the table below to reflect your decision making and share your rationales. (*Hint:* You may assign the care of a given patient to more than one person. If you do that, note the areas for which each is responsible.)

Patient	Staff Member	Task Assigned	Rationale
George Gonzalez (Room 301)			
Carrie Richards (Room 303)			
Stephanie Brown (Room 304)			
Tiffany Sheldon (Room 305)			

Copyright © 2007 by Saunders, an imprint of Elsevier Inc. All rights reserved.

7. Do you feel comfortable with your plan? Reflect on whether it was easy or difficult to accomplish.

 • Click on **Return to Nurses' Station**.
 • Visit each patient by clicking on the room number (301, 303, 304, and 305).
 • Click on **Initial Observations** and **Clinical Alerts**.
 • Take vital signs and complete a focused assessment for each patient. To do this, click on **Take Vital Signs**, **Patient Care**, and **Physical Assessment**. Note significant observations. (If you want to review feedback on your assessment, click on **Leave the Floor** and then on **Preceptor's Evaluations**.)

8. What is the purpose of making focused assessments on all assigned patients?

9. Have your priorities changed or remained the same as a result of this experience?

10. A nurse needs to anticipate changes such as new admissions, changes in patient condition, needs of parents, need to complete discharge teaching, etc. What possibilities might you anticipate in the scenarios you are facing?

Copyright © 2007 by Saunders, an imprint of Elsevier Inc. All rights reserved.

11. Given your reflection and some of the possibilities you are considering, do you wish to make any changes in your assignment? Complete a new table below. If there is no change, write "Same" in the box. Rationales should be provided for the changes you made.

Patient	Staff Member	Task Assigned	Rationale
George Gonzalez (Room 301)			
Carrie Richards (Room 303)			
Stephanie Brown (Room 304)			
Tiffany Sheldon (Room 305)			

12. What responsibilities do you have regarding care provided by the LPN?

13. What responsibilities do you have regarding care provided by the nursing assistant?

14. There is an empty bed on the unit. If there is an admission during your shift, who is responsible for the initial admission assessment and generation of a nursing care plan?

Copyright © 2007 by Saunders, an imprint of Elsevier Inc. All rights reserved.

• Now review lab work for each of your patients.
  • Click on **Chart** and then on **301**.
  • Click on and review the **Laboratory Reports** tab.
  • Repeat the two previous steps for each of your assigned patients.

15. Below, identify the lab work in which you are most interested at this point and give a rationale for your interest and/or concern.

Patient	Lab Values	Rationale
George Gonzalez (Room 301)		
Carrie Richards (Room 303)		
Stephanie Brown (Room 304)		
Tiffany Sheldon (Room 305)		

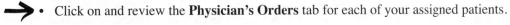

  • Click on and review the **Physician's Orders** tab for each of your assigned patients.

16. Below, rank each of your patients from the most unstable to the most stable, with 1 being the most unstable and 4 being the most stable.

	Patient	Status
_____	George Gonzalez	a. 1
_____	Carrie Richards	b. 2
_____	Stephanie Brown	c. 3
_____	Tiffany Sheldon	d. 4

Copyright © 2007 by Saunders, an imprint of Elsevier Inc. All rights reserved.

17. Discuss your choices, identifying any factors that are affecting the situation.

Exercise 2

Clinical Preparation: Writing Activity

30 minutes

- Sign in to work at Pacific View Regional Hospital for Period of Care 1. (*Note:* If you are already in the virtual hospital from a previous exercise, click on **Leave the Floor** and then **Restart the Program** to get to the sign-in window.)
- From the Patient List, select George Gonzalez (Room 301), Carrie Richards (Room 303), Stephanie Brown (Room 304), and Tiffany Sheldon (Room 305).
- Click on **Go to Nurses' Station**.
- Click on **Map** in the lower right corner of your screen.

1. Look at the physical layout of the unit. Are you satisfied with the way rooms have been assigned? Explain your answer.

2. When admitted to the hospital, each patient is admitted to Room 301, and then the charge nurse makes the actual room assignment. In the table below, assign rooms to represent your ideal configuration for these four patients.

Patient	Ideal Room Number
George Gonzalez	
Carrie Richards	
Stephanie Brown	
Tiffany Sheldon	

Copyright © 2007 by Saunders, an imprint of Elsevier Inc. All rights reserved.

3. Provide a rationale for your overall layout. What aspects of patient care did you consider?

4. What criteria would you use to make a room change?

5. Remember that changes in room assignments are not to be taken lightly. Departments need to be notified. Time of day needs to be considered. Also, there are physical aspects of the move that the nursing staff must be involved in. Given these considerations, would you make the same decision? Explain your answer.

Copyright © 2007 by Saunders, an imprint of Elsevier Inc. All rights reserved.

6. You are the nurse in charge, and you get a call that Tommy Douglas is being transferred from the ICU to the Pediatric Unit for hospice care. Where do you want to admit Tommy Douglas? Provide a rationale for your decision.

7. Who will be assigned to admit Tommy Douglas to the unit?

Congratulations! You have completed work on managing, delegating, and priority setting. Move on to the next lesson to address further scope of practice issues and application of management principles in responding to changing events.

Copyright © 2007 by Saunders, an imprint of Elsevier Inc. All rights reserved.

Pediatric Nursing Care Management: Part 2

∽ **Reading Assignment:** Review priorities of care for each of the following medical diagnoses and situations:
- Hospitalization of Children (Chapter 11, pages 288-304)
- Terminal Illness (Chapter 12, pages 320-331)
- Bronchiolitis (Chapter 21, pages 622-626)
- Diabetes Mellitus (Chapter 27, pages 898-915)
- Head Injury (Chapter 28, pages 927-931, 942-945)
- Cerebral Palsy (Chapter 28, pages 939-942)
- Meningitis (Chapter 28, pages 953-956)
- Anorexia Nervosa (Chapter 29, pages 971-975)
- Failure to Thrive (Chapter 30, pages 991-993)

Patients: George Gonzalez, Room 301
Tommy Douglas, Room 302
Carrie Richards, Room 303
Stephanie Brown, Room 304
Tiffany Sheldon, Room 305

Objectives:

- Set priorities in a given pediatric situation with a selected group of patients.
- Consider the nursing scope of practice for an RN and LPN in making assignment decisions.
- Demonstrate the ability to make effective use of ancillary personnel.
- Demonstrate effective decision making in selected pediatric situations.
- Respond to a variety of factors that affect decision making.

In this lesson you will build on the previous lesson and continue with the application of management principles in the care of five patients. Additionally, you will have the opportunity to make decisions in response to situations that can come up on the Pediatric Unit.

Copyright © 2007 by Saunders, an imprint of Elsevier Inc. All rights reserved.

Exercise 1

 CD-ROM Activity

 30 minutes

You are the taking charge of the 3-11 p.m. shift (1500-2300) on the Pediatric Unit. You have four patients: George Gonzalez, Carrie Richards, Stephanie Brown, and Tiffany Sheldon. You know that Tommy Douglas is going to be transferred from ICU and will be a hospice patient.

1. Evening shift staff members are arriving, and the supervisor is offering to send a nurse from the ICU when Tommy is transferred. There will then be two RNs, an LPN, and a nursing assistant. However, the pediatric LPN who has been scheduled will be an hour late. Given this situation, what will you do about report, assignments, and the new admission?

 • Sign in to work at Pacific View Regional Hospital for Period of Care 2. (*Note:* If you are already in the virtual hospital from a previous exercise, click on **Leave the Floor** and then **Restart the Program** to get to the sign-in window.)

• From the Patient List, select George Gonzalez (Room 301), Tommy Douglas (Room 302), Carrie Richards (Room 303), Stephanie Brown (Room 304), and Tiffany Sheldon (Room 305).

• Click on **Get Report** and read the report for each of your patients.

• Take notes to use for planning your shift.

Copyright © 2007 by Saunders, an imprint of Elsevier Inc. All rights reserved.

2. Read the report and imagine what it would be like to hear it from another nurse. (A more realistic option is to have someone read it to you.) Make a worksheet below, listing your concerns and the tasks that will need to be accomplished.

3. Review your list and determine the priorities for 4-7 p.m. (1600-1900). Remember to include meal and break times.

4. Reflect on your priority list. Does it seem workable? Is there anything you can delegate to another staff member? Explain.

Copyright © 2007 by Saunders, an imprint of Elsevier Inc. All rights reserved.

5. You anticipate that Tommy Douglas' parents will need a great deal of support and that it will be a challenge to leave his room once you begin working with them. How will you handle this situation?

Exercise 2

 ### CD-ROM Activity

 30 minutes

You are assigned to complete Tommy Douglas' admission.

• Sign in to work at Pacific View Regional Hospital for Period of Care 2. (*Note:* If you are already in the virtual hospital from a previous exercise, click on **Leave the Floor** and then **Restart the Program** to get to the sign-in window.)
• From the Patient List, select George Gonzalez (Room 301), Tommy Douglas (Room 302), Carrie Richards (Room 303), Stephanie Brown (Room 304), and Tiffany Sheldon (Room 305).
• Click on **Go to Nurses' Station** and then on **302**.
• Click on **Vital Signs** and review the readings.
• Click on **Patient Care**.
• Click on and review the **Initial Observations**.
• Click on **Physical Assessment** and complete a head-to-toe assessment.

1. Note monitoring and other equipment that is being used for Tommy Douglas.

2. Identify specific assessments that concern you at this point.

Copyright © 2007 by Saunders, an imprint of Elsevier Inc. All rights reserved.

3. Who would you assign to care for Tommy Douglas? What variables are you considering?

4. While you are completing the admission procedures, Tommy's parents seem very guarded and they watch everything you do. Tommy's mother starts to cry and says that she should have been there and maybe Tommy wouldn't have been hurt so badly. How would you respond to her?

5. You wonder whether Tommy's family wants to be alone with him. You hesitate to ask the question because you are not sure how this would affect care for other patients. What are your options?

6. How might you ask Tommy's family what they need from you? Write your response in the words you would actually use.

Copyright © 2007 by Saunders, an imprint of Elsevier Inc. All rights reserved.

7. It is time for George Gonzalez's fingerstick. You want to see how he is handling the procedure so that you can identify the learning needs he may have. However, you also feel that Tommy Douglas' parents need support. What will you do?

 • Click on **Return to Nurses' Station** and then on **301**.

• Click on **Patient Care** and then on **Physical Assessment** to complete a focused assessment of George Gonzalez.

8. As you are working with George on his blood glucose testing, the nursing assistant tells you that Carrie Richards needs Tylenol. What will you do?

9. As you are charting your nursing assessments for George Gonzalez, the nursing assistant tells you that Carrie Richards is getting worse. List in order of priority what you will need to do.

Copyright © 2007 by Saunders, an imprint of Elsevier Inc. All rights reserved.

Exercise 3

 CD-ROM Activity

 15 minutes

1. Whenever you visit Stephanie Brown, you think that her mother seems especially stressed, and you note that she is a bit terse in her communication. Identify a plan for addressing this situation.

2. There has been a rather rowdy group visiting Tiffany Sheldon. You recognize her need to see her friends but are concerned about the comfort and well-being of the other patients. How would you handle the situation?

3. When you are in Tiffany's room, you are certain that you smell marijuana. What are your options for dealing with this situation?

Congratulations! You have successfully explored a variety of situations that affect your management of pediatric patients. This exploration will help you to make decisions in your nursing practice.

Copyright © 2007 by Saunders, an imprint of Elsevier Inc. All rights reserved.